GET S

DR SHEELA NAMBIAR wears many hats. In addition to her primary profession as an obstetrician and gynaecologist, she runs a fitness programme called Training for Life in Ooty and Chennai. Certified as a fitness and lifestyle consultant from the National Association of Fitness Certification (USA), she uses fitness as an extension of her medical practice to improve the quality of women's lives and as a form of preventive care.

In her spare time, Dr Nambiar volunteers at women's and children's organizations, where she teaches spoken English and conducts workshops. Her articles on fitness appear regularly in *The Hindu*. She loves to read, trek, travel and experiment with cooking. She divides her time between Ooty and Chennai.

GET
SIZE
WISE

Training for Life
for the Indian Woman

SHEELA NAMBIAR

RUPA

Published by
Rupa Publications India Pvt. Ltd 2013
7/16, Ansari Road, Daryaganj
New Delhi 110002

Sales centres:
Allahabad Bengaluru Chennai
Hyderabad Jaipur Kathmandu
Kolkata Mumbai

While every effort has been made to verify the authenticiy of the
information contained in this book, it is not intended as a substitute
for medical consultation with a physician. The publisher and
the author are in no way liable for the use of the information
contained in this book.

ISBN: 978-81-291-2397-8

10 9 8 7 6 5 4 3 2 1

The moral right of the author has been asserted.

Typeset by Jojy Philip, New Delhi.

Printed at Thomson Press India Ltd, Faridabad

For Sara, Rhea and Samar

CONTENTS

INTRODUCTION

The doctor of the future will give no medicine, but will interest his patients in the care of human frame, in diet, and in the cause and prevention of disease.

— *Thomas Alva Edison*

I am an obstetrician and gynaecologist. Upon completing my MD in 1994, I came back to my hometown, Ooty, to share my mother's practice, which is also obstetrics. Work was a frenzied mix of surgeries, ultrasound, babies being born, and lengthy and arduous rounds at the clinic with queues of patients impatient to be seen. There was time for little else but work. My only respite was 'running'. In exercise, I found myself re-energized and de-stressed. I had involved myself in various physical activities in school in my younger days, and had often read about the benefits of fitness later in my life. At that point, however, I had little understanding of the true meaning of fitness. I was beginning to experience what exercise could do for me, both physically and emotionally. I owe my fascination for fitness to my father, who was a keen sportsman and my best critic.

When the alarm went off, I hit the snooze button twice before finally getting out of bed at 5 a.m. My surgical list started at 6 a.m. I had meant to get in a run before heading for the theatre. The night had not been uneventful. I had been called to the hospital to deliver a beautiful baby girl. I was sleep-deprived.

It was a cold, rainy morning. The scheduled caesarean was for a patient named Shameem. She was a tiny, rotund woman, 4 feet 8 inches, weighing 75 kg by the end of her pregnancy. This was her second baby. Her first pregnancy, also a caesarean, had been done elsewhere. My anaesthetist, who is extremely skilled at anaesthetic procedures, had difficulty giving Shameem spinal anaesthesia because of the swelling and fat she had accumulated over her back. Finally, we settled for general anaesthesia and I cut through the skin—a vast amount of fat and meagre muscle—to deliver her baby. It was a bawling baby boy weighing 3.5 kg.

As I sutured the various layers of her abdominal wall, I wished I could cut away her fat and save her the trouble of trying to lose it, which I hoped she would do in the coming months.

The remaining surgical procedures—a hysterectomy, laparoscopic procedures, a few other minor procedures—went smoothly. We were out of the theatre by 10.30 a.m. After a quick breakfast of home-made multigrain bread, eggs and fruit, I had to be back in the outpatient clinic to face the rest of the morning.

My first patient was a well-heeled, elegant 50-year-old with intolerable menopausal symptoms. She needed counselling, reassurance, lifestyle changes and exercise. There were tears and expressions of 'I can't take it any more, I didn't know menopause could be so awful.' I tried to reassure her. More tears. Family issues, mother-daughter problems, a truant daughter-in-law. It went on. My nurse looked at me reproachfully: I had a waiting room full of patients to attend to.

The morning drew on. There was a village woman with breast cancer. The daughter was distraught. How could she have missed such an advanced stage of the disease? Why hadn't the mother alerted someone, or come to the hospital earlier? Why hadn't they come for the **preventive health check-ups** that were long overdue? I had seen the mother 5 years before and taught her to do the self-examination of the breast, according to her records. She had either not done it at all, or had been too scared to report the breast lump, which had now progressed to a more advanced disease. It was heartbreaking.

Then, an obese 40-year-old with an incisional hernia, who had been advised surgery. I convinced her that she needed to lose some weight first, as part of the problem was the massive amount of abdominal fat she had accumulated. Her hernia repair was bound to be unsuccessful otherwise.

Pregnant patients in varying stages of pregnancy. Postnatal patients with their babies, some wanting to know how to get back in shape, insisting their mothers overfed them and refused to allow them exercise. Some overwrought young mothers unable to handle new motherhood with postnatal depression. Patients with infertility, anxious to conceive, with overbearing mothers-in-law and nervous husbands. Over-demanding patients, hard to please. Gentle, unassuming women with life stories that would put any illustrious autobiography to shame. Women from all social and economic backgrounds.

The outpatient clinic finally came to an end at a half past two.

I had to teach a body conditioning class at 3 p.m. I just about made it after eating some cheese and my revitalizer tonic of beetroot, carrot and apple juice. It was a 45-minute session of weight training, own-body weight exercises, stretches and a lot of fun and laughter.

After a bowl of oats porridge with flaxseed powder, a fruit and milk (I always kept cooked oats in the fridge), I was ready for the rest of the day, feeling completely energized after the workout.

Back in the hospital, there was a stream of things to attend to. Patients in labour. Discharges of inpatients, ultrasound, talking to nurses, meetings and paperwork.

It was 7 p.m. by the time I managed to get in a run—30 minutes on my treadmill. My Labrador eyed me looking suitably hurt. I had missed taking him for his walk or at least a drive in the car! Dinner, a chat with my mother and then on to reading and writing into the night. As I crawled into bed close to 11 p.m., I set my alarm for 5 a.m. to go for my bike ride. I could only hope I would not be woken up again at night... Drifting off to sleep, I thought about my day. So many of the women I had attended to needed to fit regular exercise into their day. **Their lives would be so different, more productive and less filled with physical and emotional pain. All these women needed a clear, well-defined option for exercise.**

I made a decision to teach fitness and preventive care as an extension of my medical practice. It had to be more accessible even to the poorest patient with back pain, depression or just plain obesity. We already had antenatal and postnatal classes going, so why not more focused fitness sessions for non-pregnant women?

Initially I gave advice and counselled patients across the table in my consulting room. I told them to exercise and eat healthy as most doctors do. There were the women who had genuine organic problems and there were those who had problems that had arisen due to their own lifestyle choices. Obesity, back and knee pain, depression, indigestion, constipation, myalgia, diabetes, hypertension, high cholesterol levels, the list was endless. Most of these women were looking for solutions with a prescription across the table from their doctor. It did not occur to them that they were in part responsible for their ailment and could also be a part of the treatment.

I soon figured that just dialogue wasn't sufficient. **I had to walk the talk.** This required me to actually take a step into fitness professionally, obtain certification as a **fitness and lifestyle consultant** and begin with teaching group classes. It hadn't occurred to me till I actually went through the certification process, that fitness was such a vast and extremely interesting subject. The books, videos, exercises, projects, exams reminded me of going back to college all over again! It was well worth the effort, however. As a doctor, one tends to believe one knows everything about the human body. In medical college, however, we are taught about the healthy or unwell human body, not the exercising one. We do not learn how to train it, physically challenge it, and identify muscle imbalances and improper physical functionality.

It was a new and exciting experience. Teaching fitness is not the same as being a doctor. One cannot write a prescription and walk away. You had to actually see it interpreted and acted upon. A client, unlike a patient, is a very different kettle of fish! She most likely does not want to listen to you because you are asking her to do some very demanding things of her body. Instead of giving her a list of pills to swallow to make her feel better, you are, in essence, making her uncomfortable, breathless, flushed in the face, and telling her that she had to keep doing it!

When I started teaching fitness in the year 2000, the concept of aerobics or aerobic dance was alien to a majority of the women in Ooty. Moving to music was only done at parties and that too never to break sweat, lest, God forbid, you ruin your make-up. However, very soon, it became popular, even fashionable, and I continued to teach for 10 long years.

After managing to cope with my medical practice and teaching a class 6 days a week, I finally changed strategy to avoid burn-out and started my own programme, calling it **Training for Life** or **TFL**. I trained people to teach the classes for me, opened a fitness studio in Chennai, and made it into an ancillary career. An enjoyable one at that.

I spend one week in every 4–6 weeks in my studio in Chennai where I restrict myself to being a fitness and lifestyle consultant. I give my practice a break! While in Chennai, I teach, train, take classes, consult, counsel and run my studio. I give talks to corporate women on the importance of holistic wellness and conduct workshops.

While in Ooty, I run the hospital, practise obstetrics and gynaecology, consult, counsel, operate, deliver babies, and also teach fitness classes and conduct workshops with women's groups on health and wellness. As a part of the TFL programme's social module for wellness, the TFL members visit village women to talk to them on health and preventive care, and in return learn from them and their ingenious ways of survival. We have a Movie and Book Club (affectionately called the M&B Club) where we read, watch and discuss books and movies of different genres as part of the intellectual and creative aspect of wellness that we propagate at TFL.

My life is crazy, hectic and sometimes overwhelming, and although I sometimes ask myself, 'Do I really need this?' I must admit, it is thoroughly satisfying. **Obstetrics is my profession and fitness my passion.**

How do I manage both? I am not sure! It was a conscious decision to include fitness as an extension of my medical practice. I felt it was necessary as a form of preventive care and greatly complemented my medical training, and vice versa.

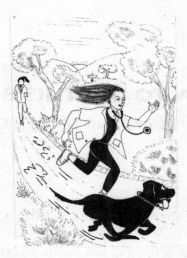

I am humbled even more by the complexity of the human body. I marvel at just how much abuse it withstands! I am thrilled at seeing how it can repair itself of myriad ailments that are most often self-imposed. I believe very strongly in the strength of a woman.

I believe we are capable of truly remarkable accomplishments; of helping and healing ourselves just as we help family and friends around us. I believe we are capable of many, many things at any age if we so much as set our mind to it! I also believe that for this to happen we need to do three things:

- Stop believing we are the victims of circumstances.
- **Understand exactly what it takes** to make the necessary changes in our lives that will benefit us. Try not to indiscriminately believe everything we hear, read or are expected to.
- **Make the necessary changes**, commitments and compromises to take steps in the right direction to better our health, without expecting instant solutions.

HOW TO USE THIS BOOK

TFL AND THE ART AND SCIENCE OF FITNESS

The best-kept secret in the fitness industry is that there is no secret!

This book does not give you any miracle cure to trim your waist, or magic exercises to obtain slim thighs. It just tells you everything that you should be doing. If done right, your waist will get trimmer and thighs slimmer, but really, there is nothing mysterious about it. It is just science and common sense.

In this book, I have tried to do two things:

- Explain and clarify that fitness includes more than just walking or dieting or doing yoga or just any one thing. It requires an adherence to the **4 pillars of fitness**.
- Clarify that every woman requires something that is uniquely suitable for her body. The same woman will also have different needs during the course of her life as she faces varied physical and emotional challenges.

This book is primarily based on scientific research, not anecdotal evidence or armchair speculation. There are hundreds of studies about health and fitness. Many are published in popular magazines. Are they to be taken seriously? How is the layperson to know? I have, to the best of my ability, filtered the hype from genuine information and knowledge and laid down some basic principles on fitness that can be followed.

HOW TO USE THE BOOK

- Focus on the **4 major pillars of fitness, nutrition, rest and attitude**. I believe understanding these is essential to make informed decisions about your own health and wellness.
- My first chapter 'Does Weight Matter?' was conceived and placed as the opening chapter simply to address women's common misconceptions about weight and size.
- Most of the chapters have a combination of Quick Facts columns, DIYs (Do It Yourself) and other tables for ease of reference at the end.
- There are sample charts in some chapters and the appendices, that you could fill in to keep track of your own progress.
- There are sample exercise routines in some chapters for your reference. Please note that these are only samples, and are not universally applicable. One needs to be guided through routines.
- I have deliberately not included photographs of exercises in this book not only for want of space but also because this book is primarily about understanding what you need to know about fitness in general, not about specific exercises.

Once you have acquired a basic working knowledge of fitness and your bodies, you will not succumb easily to mindless myths, the media frenzy created by a latest fitness craze, or a weight loss mantra.

> You will learn to listen to your own bodies and understand them at a level deeper than that of the lure of the weighing scale or mirror.

I have also drawn greatly from my own experience with women in general and women in training. I have applied what seems to work on a practical level **for the Indian woman**. She works under a different kind of psychological pressure.

Women have to learn to become autonomous in their decision-making regarding their life choices, their health and wellness. They can then be confident of not falling for the usual marketing pitch of a savvy salesman selling dreams of a perfect body. They can look forward to making fitness a lifelong journey not just a passing phase with a constrained objective like 'lose 10 kg'.

CHAPTER 1

DOES WEIGHT MATTER?

THE MISLEADING SCALE AND OUR OBSESSION WITH IT

In the Middle Ages, they had guillotines, stretch racks, whips and chains. Nowadays, we have a much more effective torture device called the bathroom scale.

—*Stephen Philips*

Stepping on the scale seems to be a preoccupation for many dieters and fitness enthusiasts. Scales are everywhere: at the bathroom, the gym, the health club, the doctor's office. I have even noticed people in gyms approaching the scale with some apprehension and perhaps a few muttered prayers every day before *and* after their workout. Despite this fixation with weight on the scale we seem to be getting fatter than ever.

The number indicated on the scale is rarely a good indicator of what our body consists of. Weight on the scale alone cannot tell you anything about the distribution of that weight. It does not take into account the ratio of fat to muscle tissue. This can cause very lean but muscular individuals to assume they are fatter than they really are, and people, who perhaps weigh within the normal range but who have a high fat percentage, to believe mistakenly that they are doing just fine.

'Oh my God, I have gained 2 kg!' is the squeal of agony you hear on the gym floor from women obsessed with that magical number. Women have been literally brainwashed into believing that they have to be of a certain weight. We learn at a very early age that we have to maintain our figures.

I still recall stepping on the weighing scale in school with bated breath during the monthly weighing-in session, or during the pre-sports day assessment. Nothing else was evaluated, just one's height and weight. Many kids are exposed to some form of exercise in school. Most of what they are taught is unscientific. There are the athletes and the non-athletes. The non-athletes sit on the sidelines and cheer the athletes during matches and inter-school athletic games. They have no hope of being taken seriously on the field. One is not really taught fitness from a holistic perspective. Neither is it ingrained in youth that fitness is related to health and wellness for their future and is not just a reflection of how high you jump or how fast you run in school.

It is no wonder then that women, upon growing older, approach fitness with a certain concealed anxiety. Their perception of exercise comes from their school days, from magazines telling them that they need to exercise in order to look a certain way, or from their doctors pronouncing ominous warnings concerning their health unless they start exercising.

> Weight is only one aspect of overall fitness. I believe we also need to stop looking at exercise purely as a means to an end, that is, weight loss. Weight loss is only a by-product, a very gratifying one, no doubt.

Being within your expected weight range is very important from a health perspective for several reasons. To drive home the importance of staying within the recommended weight, here are some research findings:

- We all know obesity can lead to heart disease, diabetes, high blood pressure, high cholesterol, gall stones, and breast, colon and endometrial (uterine) cancer.
- Brain scans on obese people have found that their brain volume is less than that of normally weighing individuals, who appeared much older than their slimmer counterparts.
- Obesity is related to depression and mood disorders.
- Obese individuals are at a higher risk of fall and injury, due to lack of balance and reduced strength of muscles in addition to the excess fat.
- Obesity is often associated with various skin conditions like fungal infections, folliculitis, cellulitis, and bacterial infections of the skin called erythrasma occurring due to sweat in the skin folds.
- Obesity has been found to impair sleep. Sleep apnoea, which is a condition where individuals actually stop breathing in their sleep, is more common in the obese.
- Obesity reduces the quality of life in general and studies have shown a remarkable improvement in the quality of life following weight loss.
- Obesity has been found to be closely related to poor self-esteem in both adults and children.

So, you start exercising because you need to lose weight. Ask yourself this question: after you lose the proposed weight, then what?

Do you stop working out because you have achieved your goal? How do you plan to persist with your fitness, if at all? Most women who have achieved their weight loss goals, or who are already slim mistakenly believe that exercise need not feature in their lives.

If we de-focus from **weight** to just **fitness**, **how we feel and live**, and most importantly our **quality of life**, our chances of persevering with a fitness routine that evolves and grows with us is greater. It also helps us enjoy fitness (is that even a possibility, you ask?), yes, enjoy fitness, to the extent where it is not just an hour one spends sweating it out as an obsessive means to some cosmetic end, but also a journey of self-discovery, a source of pleasure, even delight.

> Losing weight on the scale alone without altering body composition (fat to muscle ratio) by losing body fat percentage can actually be detrimental to health, especially if it is at the expense of losing muscle.

WEIGHT LOSS WITH DIET ALONE

You could most certainly lose weight if you starve yourself or go on an extreme calorie-deficient diet. Many women do just that. Somehow, it appears that they seem to consider it easier and more effective than working out. I have spent many hours listening to women justify their futile and ridiculous diets. It seems appealing to them to choose to crash-diet rather than sweat it out at the gym.

IS THERE A FAMINE?

When you go on a starvation diet where the calories consumed are clearly not sufficient even to sustain basic

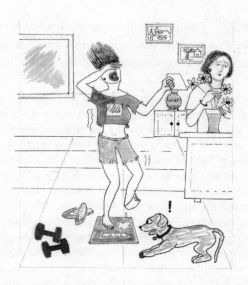

body metabolism, muscle is also broken down to provide for energy. The body feels there is a famine and lowers its metabolic rate accordingly and manages to survive on minimum calories. This was a survival instinct for the caveman when food was scarce and the next meal was never truly guaranteed. These days, with our abundant culinary choices, this is hardly the case. When you go off that dreadful diet, which you will invariably need to, as it is not life-sustainable, your body remains accustomed to surviving on a very low-calorie intake. If you then proceed to attempt to eat anywhere near normal, much to your exasperation, the extra calories are stored as fat. Defeats the whole purpose of the diet and the struggle doesn't it?

This seems to me like self-sabotage. So why do women persist with it believing that stringent, inflexible diets with bizarre food combinations will work for them? That drastic weight loss is the only answer? Perhaps because they want to get into that sexy little blouse for a cousin's wedding as early as next week. There is no time for workouts, meal-planning and laborious counselling sessions. They want to lose weight immediately.

Monisha was significantly overweight. She had been this way all her life. For as long as I can remember she had struggled with various diets, her weight yo-yoing, torturing herself by eating strange combinations of food, or restricting herself to liquids, and so on. Once she went to a nature cure resort where they made her live on cucumber juice and mudbaths. It was frightfully expensive, but by the time she got out in 2 weeks' time she was thrilled to be a few kilos lighter. She had got her money's worth, hadn't she?

Well, of course, she went right back to her original weight! It is all very well to take drastic measures like these non-life-sustaining practices to lose some weight. You will, but that's just the point. They are not practical in the real world. You can't wallow in mud in the hope of drawing impurities or water out of your body and neither can you sustain yourself on meagre amounts of food or water.

Then she discovered Lasix, the diuretic. She developed a high blood pressure (of course she did!), and part of the medication included a small dose of Lasix to control the blood pressure. To her delight, she found that when she took the drug, she was not only lighter, but also managed to get into a blouse she couldn't get into earlier. Joy oh joy!

My conversations with her used to always leave me feeling frustrated. Her cheerful nature and seeming acceptance of her weight were beguiling. Only we knew her constant war with herself. She always expressed sheer amazement, even shock at anyone who had significantly lost weight and become fit on exercise and a healthy eating plan. It was as if the impossible was being divulged.

'You can also do it,' I would encourage her. 'But it requires a lifestyle change, an understanding of food and a commitment to...

...regular exercise, not random attempts at weight loss using the most unsavoury methods.' She laughed with me at herself. That was what was most charming about her!

Finally, she did get on an exercise programme, and has managed to lose weight. More importantly, she feels wonderful, she tells me. Her fitness levels have improved immensely. She has actually begun to enjoy working out, provided, she says, it is in a class with other people, to music with dance moves, and so on.

Each to her own. Not many women can train without constant encouragement or companionship. If that is your concern, you should join a motivating group class, where you are guided properly.

I suspect, most women do understand this concept of healthy, balanced eating but are too lazy to analyse their food choices and want to be instructed as to what to eat and, more importantly, what not to eat. That way, responsibility can be transferred to the dietician concerned.

The long-term consequences of losing weight rapidly and on a very low-calorie diet alone are, however, not attractive and, invariably, the weight lost comes right back with interest! The weight you lose in this way is mostly muscle mass, and you certainly don't want that if you know what's good for you. You also lose your hair, your nails, your healthy skin, not to mention your sunny personality and even your ability to have a productive day as you obsess about food.

Some studies have found that severe dieting and cycles of weight loss followed by weight gain can be detrimental to health. Drastic changes in body weight following yo-yo dieting could, in itself, affect the blood pressure, cholesterol and the heart. The very purpose of losing weight, which is to improve health, is then defeated. This does not mean that overweight and obese individuals should not try to lose fat. They should be encouraged to do so in a healthy and scientific manner with **exercise and a balanced diet**, not starvation diets alone.

> Extreme low-calorie diets cause one to lose muscle mass along with fat. The result may be a smaller body, but one that remains flabby in the same shape as the earlier fat one and, worse, with less muscle.

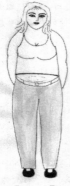

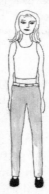

Excess Fat   Only Diet

The key, then, is eating a healthy balanced diet, and introducing the right amount of exercise to maintain and increase your muscle mass, while losing fat. This has to be a **lifestyle** rather than a fad one follows for a couple of weeks in the hope of quick weight loss.

The weighing scale therefore has gained a great degree of needless significance. Don't get me wrong. It is definitely an easy way to assess your **total weight**. As long as you understand what that means and use it to your advantage, you can hold on to your weighing scale.

The weight on the scale is a combination of:
- Water weight

- Fat weight
- Muscle weight
- Weight of our bones
- Weight of organs, the brain, etc.

When we address weight loss, what we need to essentially concentrate on is fat weight. We certainly should not be losing muscle, bone or any other form of weight.

It has been found that losing weight and maintaining that weight loss is next to impossible for many individuals. Blame it on genetics, the environment, hormones or viral gene mutation; these individuals are somehow unable to sustain weight loss over long periods of time. In such circumstances, it is better to focus on fitness levels rather than weight alone. From a health perspective, fitness levels are far more important. Focusing on fitness levels and not fixating about the scale, rather than giving up on exercise altogether because of only a marginal change in weight, allows such women to achieve a better health status.

WEIGHT LOSS AND AGEING

Every now and then I meet older women who are thrilled that they have managed to maintain their weight on the scale over the years despite **not working out at all!** Something they appear to be particularly proud of. There are two problems with this:

- Weight loss is **not** the only benefit of working out. A woman, pleased that she has not gained or lost weight without exercise, is not doing herself any favours. If she is not or has not been exercising, she is not experiencing the multitude of other benefits of exercise like greater productivity, better mood, protection for her bones and heart, and so on.

- Since the weight on the scale is indicative of the composite body weight and since they have not been exercising to build muscle mass, these women are, in all likelihood, losing muscle due to disuse, and gaining fat, thereby maintaining weight on the scale. This is not an accomplishment to be particularly delighted with. Changing the body composition for the worse—more fat, less muscle—cannot benefit you in any way.

The solution then is to start training with weights to build muscle. This is particularly important for older women. Weight training has another very important benefit for older women—**protection from osteoporosis.**

With age and falling oestrogen levels, women do tend to gain fat. Moreover, the distribution of the fat differs from that of a younger woman. It accumulates over the abdomen and upper part of the hips. The gluteal (buttock) and leg muscles become smaller (atrophy) and the lower body tends to appear thinner, while the waist begins to look suspiciously wider even if the woman is slim overall. Women also tend to lose bone as they age and this in turn makes them lighter on the scale. Interestingly, it seems as if menopause mimics this metabolic syndrome with a tendency to similar changes in weight, fat distribution, elevated LDL cholesterol, and a propensity for diabetes and heart disease. The female hormones protect the women largely from these changes. Once we stop secreting these hormones after menopause, it is our responsibility to protect ourselves from these ailments with lifestyle efforts like:

- Regular aerobic exercise to keep the heart and respiratory system healthy and fat percentage optimum.
- Inclusion of heart-healthy food in our diet, cutting down sugar and saturated fats.
- Training with weights to increase deteriorating muscle mass.

- Improving flexibility to keep the muscle supple, and so on.

CAUSES OF WEIGHT LOSS

Losing weight on the scale could mean a number of things, all not necessarily beneficial to health or fitness:

Diseases: Some of the more alarming reasons women sometimes lose weight drastically and suddenly could be due to diseases like **diabetes**, **hyperthyroidism** or, worse still, a **cancer.** If you are losing weight for no apparent reason, do have a medical evaluation to determine the cause.

Drugs: Some drugs can cause weight loss, at least in the initial stages. The newer antidepressants and drugs for hypothyroidism, diabetes and polycystic ovaries, may cause you to lose some weight. The weight usually stabilizes with the continued use of the drug.

Stress: Some women tend to lose weight when under extreme stress. They often lose their appetite, eat less and burn more calories with worrying. This weight is not all fat, but includes muscle mass, which once again is not advisable. Of course, at the other end of the spectrum, stress can cause weight gain for some women due to mindless eating, and the lack of sleep and exercise. It all depends on how your body responds to stress.

Muscle loss: It could mean that you have lost muscle mass. Muscle, being lean tissue, for the same volume weighs more than fat. Losing a little muscle therefore can reflect significantly on the scale as weight loss. Muscle is lost with prolonged disuse and age.

Bone loss: Losing weight on the scale could also mean you are losing bone. As we age, bones de-mineralize and become lighter, more fragile and susceptible to breakage. Older women, who have not maintained their bone and muscle mass with regular weight training, are therefore frail and lighter on the scale. Many of them, of course, manage to maintain and even increase the fat percentage in their body over the years and balance the scale pretty well!

Water loss: It could also indicate water loss from the cells of the body. Ever noticed the scales dip after an acute episode of a gastrointestinal upset like food poisoning, traveller's diarrhoea or shigellosis? This is the result of the water lost from our gut. Similarly, sitting in a sauna or in extreme heat leading to excessive sweating can also result in weight loss on the scale. Sixty per cent of our body is water. We can lose water in the form of sweat and excrement.

Fever: Soon after an episode of illness, you may find, to your delight I am sure, that you have lost some weight on the scale. This is essentially water that you have depleted as a result of the elevated body temperature that we recognize as a fever.

Weight cutting, which is a concept sometimes practised by athletes, involves reduction in body weight just before a sporting or athletic event. It is achieved by the use of diuretics, laxatives, inducing excessive sweating in the sauna, by wrapping the body in polythene and other ingenious ways. Athletes participate in such practices to put their lighter bodies at an advantage in their sport.

Water is dynamic and often we find we have retained some extra water in our bodies causing the feet and face to swell. This happens with sudden changes in altitude or weather. There could also be some amount of **water retention** resulting in premenstrual bloating in some women. Young women complaining that they become fat just before their period often besiege me. Water retention is due to the hormonal flux in your system during the cycle. Some women appear to respond more severely to the cyclical female hormones oestrogen and progesterone.

> An interesting use of this dynamic property of the water in our body is the application of heated body wraps and electrical stimulators to facilitate drawing water out from the superficial cells of the body through the skin, in 'Slimming Parlours'.
>
> The hypothesis is that you are **melting fat!** Do you see any fat oozing out of your skin? Better still, **mobilizing fat**. To go where? Into your bloodstream to clog the arteries? It is astonishing what women will believe!
>
> No doubt one may see a marginal decrease in the circumference of the body part that is so wrapped, or weight loss on the scale. Essentially, water loss. This comes right back within 24 hours.
>
> This is a clever assault on the psyche and intelligence of women: the promise of quick and easy weight loss while one lies in comfort watching TV.

Since all of these variables (muscle mass, bone and water) can show up as weight loss on the scale, you can now understand why it is so important to evaluate what exactly it is that you have lost before celebrating.

Fundamentally, what you need to lose is fat: the fat that is inside the abdomen covering vital organs, and the fat surrounding and encasing the muscles, just beneath the surface of the skin. Obviously, you cannot and should not lose all the fat. There is a baseline and normal range of fat percentage that is allowed and required at various ages. Staying within those guidelines is more important than weighing oneself innumerable times with the hope of losing a few grams.

Karina had what I called scale mania. She actually stood on the scale before and after her workout every day! She looked perfectly slim, weighed 55 kg, which on her 5'3" frame was perfectly acceptable according to height/weight charts. She was to get married in 3 months and claimed she wanted to lose 5 kg.

'From where?' I asked her, 'Your eyelashes?'

I tried to explain to her the importance of fat percentage, the redundancy of the scale, especially in her case, and to make her see that all she needed to do was build muscle so she could be in better shape.

'Muscle?' she squealed, 'But that will make me heavy, doesn't muscle weigh more than fat?' Well, at least she got that right!

There was no dissuading her. She was a Cardio Queen. Her cardio lasted easily more than an hour. Despite the trainers admonishing her and telling her she had done enough, she would actually sneak back on the treadmill for another 15 minutes before leaving, much to the absolute horror of the other clients! She refused to lift more than 2 kg for any exercise while weight-training, which was unavoidable, claiming it was too heavy when it was clearly not. It came to a point where I was worried she was getting anorexic. I had to tell her to stop. She sulked.

Then she fell ill. A mild viral infection. It left her completely drained and unable to come to the gym, for which I was thankful! I suspect it was because she had put her body under undue stress, resulting in lowered immunity. By the time of her wedding, she had lost quite a lot of weight and looked almost emaciated. I joked with her that she need never have come to the gym at all; all she needed was to fall ill!

I never saw her again until after her wedding. She turned up with her husband 6 months later, looking happy, and...a little sheepish.

Her husband, it appears, is a bodybuilder! Appalled by her lack of weight training, he had decided he would take matters into his own hands and insisted she come back to train properly.

'He says it doesn't matter how slim I am because I am flabby,' she pouted.

Hmmm. I had told her that many months ago! Obviously, it hadn't registered too well.

She came back and trained sensibly. She built some muscle, cut down on her cardio, incorporated stretches regularly, looked great, and was surprised that she actually felt absolutely terrific.

'I was in fact tired a lot, earlier,' she confessed. 'All I wanted to do after working out was sleep!' That was fundamentally because she was not doing what her body required. Instead, she was impelling it to do what she thought she needed, to achieve a slimmer silhouette. **She was not listening to her body.**

Her husband on the other hand had to be initiated into doing some cardio! Although he didn't train in my gym, he would come in often and discuss the merits and demerits of doing cardio. He wanted to look 'beefed up' (his words) and if he did cardio he would get too lean, wouldn't he?

'So what is the difference between you and Karina?' I asked him. 'She focused on cardio, and you on weight training. Either one, to the exclusion of the other, cannot produce the best results. Do you just want to be "beefed up", and then collapse with a heart attack, or would you rather live longer, looking great?'

Karina tells me he has started running 3 times a week.

This story teaches us two things:
- Weight on the scale is not the only priority if you want a healthy body.
- Learn to listen to your body when it implores you to stop being foolish by overtraining, training wrong, or not training at all.

WHAT ARE THE THINGS ABOUT YOUR BODY YOU NEED TO KEEP IN MIND?

- Height/weight charts
- BMI or Body Mass Index
- Girth measurements of various parts of the body
- Waist hip ratio

Height/Weight Charts

Typical height/weight charts can also be misleading, where an athlete, for instance, may be overweight going solely by the scale and standard charts, but could have a body fat percentage well within or even below the normal. Athletes, people who train with weights, and bodybuilders have a higher muscle mass and could weigh more than they look.

A young woman may weigh well within the norm of the height/weight charts, and may even look very slim, but could possibly have an accumulation of excess fat thereby leaving her falsely reassured, but unfit and flabby.

So, do we do away with height/weight charts? Not necessarily. They can be used keeping everything in perspective. The normal range or weight as indicated in the height/weight chart is a broad guideline to indicate where we stand. In addition to the weighing scale, which I suspect is not going anywhere in a hurry, we need to apply fat percentages and girth measures to get a better idea of the **content** of our body—**fat** or **muscle**.

Standard Height and Weight for Indian Men and Women
(Courtesy: LIC of India)

Height (Feet/m)	Men Weight (kg)	Women Weight (kg)
5' 0" (1.523 m)	50.8-54.4	50.8-54.4
5' 1" (1.548 m)	51.7-55.3	51.7-55.3
5' 2" (1.574 m)	56.3-60.3	53.1-56.7
5' 3" (1.599 m)	57.6-61.7	54.4-58.1
5' 4" (1.624 m)	58.9-63.5	56.3-59.9
5' 5" (1.650 m)	60.8-65.3	57.6-61.2
5' 6" (1.675 m)	62.2-66.7	58.9-63.5
5' 7" (1.700 m)	64.0-68.5	60.8-65.3

Height (Feet/m)	Men Weight (kg)	Women Weight (kg)
5' 8" (1.726 m)	65.8-70.8	62.2-66.7
5' 9" (1.751 m)	67.6-72.6	64.0-68.5
5' 10" (1.777 m)	69.4-74.4	65.8-70.3
5' 11" (1.802 m)	71.2-76.2	67.1-71.7
6' 0" (1.827 m)	73.0-78.5	68.5-73.9
6' 1" (1.853 m)	73.3-80.7	73.3-80.7
6' 2" (1.878 m)	77.6-83.5	77.6-83.5
6' 3" (1.904 m)	79.8-85.9	79.8-85.9

BMI—BODY MASS INDEX

BMI is evaluated using your height and weight. On account that the formula uses only height and weight and not specifically the fat percentage, its value is limited to broadly categorizing individuals into underweight, normal weight, overweight and obese categories. This helps assess disease risk. To assess improvement in body composition, fat loss or muscle gain, however, BMI is ineffective.

BMI is calculated using the following formula:
Weight in kilograms/Height in metres squared
(To convert inches to metres, multiply by 0.0254; to convert pounds to kilograms, divide by 2.2)

INTERNATIONAL VALUES FOR BMI

BMI	Disease Risk	Classification
< 20.00	Moderate to very high	Underweight
20.00-21.99	Low	Acceptable
22.00-24.00	Very low	
25.00-26.99	Low	Overweight
27.00-29.99	Moderate	
30.00-39.99	High	Obese
> 40.00	Very High	

BMI can be used widely to determine if you are within a normal range. Keep in mind, however, that it uses weight alone and not the body fat percentage to evaluate the disease risk and classification. BMI can be used in conjunction with the body fat percentage and waist hip ratio to assess your overall health status and risk for disease.

In an interesting study done in Mysore, it was found that, among Indians, diabetes was prevalent even with a BMI of 23–25, and an average waist circumference of 81–90 cm which is considered normal by Western standards. Obviously, as Indians we are at a greater risk of developing Type 2 diabetes and we don't necessarily need to fall into the obese category, or reach a certain waist girth to achieve this! **In the Indian scenario** alarm bells should sound when the BMI is over 23 (as opposed to the global value of 25 being the cut-off according to the health ministry of India and other organizations).

BMI	Indian Standards
> 23	Overweight
>25	Obese
>32.5	May require bariatric surgery!

However, in August 2000, Dr C. Everett Koop of Shape Up America! issued an advisory stating that one's body fat percentage is superior to the currently accepted body mass index (BMI), as a measure of healthy weight.

GIRTH MEASURES

The humble inch tape is of enormous value to assess fat loss in specific areas. When you lose fat, you may find that it disappears from certain areas in your body more easily than others. Your arms may decrease in circumference but your thighs may remain the same initially. Where and how your body loses fat is genetically predetermined.

A standardized method of measuring the waist, which has been used in population studies in India, is through the midway point between the lowest rib and the upper edge of the iliac (hip) bone on the side of the waist. Some women's navels may be higher or fat accumulation may make it appear lower on the abdomen. To avoid these problems, measure midway between the rib and hip bone.

Alternately, have your own two or three standard measures between the lower border of the rib cage and upper border of the hip bone to assess progressive fat loss. Measure your waist in three different areas:

- The smallest circumference (just beneath the ribcage)
- At the navel
- Below the navel

Keep a record of these values taken over a period of time to assess your fat loss. A slim waist and flat stomach is a clear indicator of lowering fat percentage in the body.

You can also keep a record of other girth measurements in your food and exercise journal. Measurements need to be taken at various points, preferably by the same examiner or yourself to avoid inter-observer variations. (See Appendix V for what the Body Statistics chart should look like.)

Changes in girth measurements without changes in body weight are significant. Body fat percentage evaluation will reveal the whole picture. A girth chart is extremely useful to monitor fat loss and its progress. It is common to get disheartened when you do not see the expected change in the weighing scale. Correlate with the girth chart.

If you find you are declining in girth, but perhaps not losing much on the scale, it is an indication of muscle gain. This is a good thing.

WAIST MEASURE AND WAIST HIP RATIO

Simply measuring your waistline can help you not only assess your health risk but also give you some idea if you are losing fat. Fat accumulating inside the abdominal cavity is called **visceral fat** (around the vital organs) and that on the surface of the abdominal wall is called **subcutaneous fat**. Visceral fat accumulation is the most dangerous, and endangers your health by releasing inflammatory substances and magnifies the risk to diabetes by increasing insulin resistance.

Measure your waist. It is the single most important assessment you can do to keep your health in check. Any value above 80 cm for Indian women—at the level of the navel—is to be regarded with great concern. Try and keep the value below 72 cm.

The waist hip ratio can also be used to assess an individual's health risk. It is calculated as the waist circumference divided by the hip circumference. Measure the waist at the narrowest point and the hip at the widest and the ratio of the two, denoted by a decimal number, is categorized in the chart below:

WAIST IN CENTIMETRES/HIP IN CENTIMETRES

0.8 or below	Low risk
0.81-0.85	Moderate risk
Above 0.85	High risk

PLEASANTLY PLUMP!

At the other end of the spectrum, amazingly, I find that being slim, thin or lean is sometimes frowned upon, especially by older women in Indian society. Women are encouraged to remain plump which they view as an indicator of attractiveness, health and affluence. Obviously, in poorer communities, being plump or overweight is associated with affluence and easy access to adequate food, whereas a malnourished, thin woman would be seen as poor, and that is somehow understandable. What is not, is this idea that being plump, even fat, is essentially an indication of health. Steady weight gain, especially after marriage and childbirth, is acceptable and even encouraged. Many young women I know diet secretly to maintain or lose weight, as they are not allowed to exercise. They resort to desperate measures like starving themselves in the hope of staying slim.

With the abundance of food choices available, women seeking to lose weight should exercise regularly and eat a balanced diet rather than resort to torturing their bodies with unhealthy practices.

GAINING WEIGHT THE HEALTHY WAY

On the flip side, I know of several women who wish to gain weight. They are the skinny ones, often self-conscious about being flat-chested, and considered weak. If it was just weight on the scale that is needed to be gained, consuming a large number of calories, from your favourite high-fat foods like ice creams, chocolates, French fries, kheer, etc., and leading a sedentary lifestyle over a period of time is all that is required. These women will eventually gain enough fat to look larger. Obviously, this is not a sensible approach. What is required is to build muscle. This does not automatically happen by consuming an increased number of calories. To gain muscle one needs to actually train the muscle against resistance.

> *You need to gain weight by building muscle, not adding fat!*

Before setting out to start training, even these slim women need to have their fat percentage assessed. They may be surprised that despite appearing thin, their fat percentage may be more than it should. Training to gain muscle is hard work. It requires dedicated training with weights and consuming a very balanced and nutritious diet that is adequate in protein. It also requires commitment and perseverance because muscle gain does not happen overnight.

These women are called **hard gainers**. Every one of us is endowed with a certain amount of muscle and a certain number of muscle fibres. In order to increase muscle mass, these fibres have to increase in size. This happens when we challenge the muscle beyond its normal capacity. For example when the shoulder muscle, the deltoid, which is not accustomed to anything beyond lifting clothes off a hanger or occasionally picking up your kids, is put through 3-4 sets of shoulder presses and lat raises, the muscles are shocked into increasing in size and recruiting more fibres to cope with the demand of the exercise.

SIZE OF THE BREAST

I would, at this point like to make a mention of breast size. The female breast is mainly fatty tissue. When you lose fat all over the body by consuming less and exercising more, you will lose fat from the breast as well. You cannot direct your body not to lose breast fat alone. Neither can you guide it to lose specifically from that area as from any other area. **That is, spot reduction does not work.**

You can increase the strength and size of the pectoral muscle lying beneath the breast tissue, but you cannot specifically increase or decrease its size. Pregnancy and breastfeeding can increase the size of your breasts. Once the woman stops breastfeeding, it usually goes back to the pre-pregnancy size.

The size of the breast seems to cause undue concern for many women. I have even had women stop exercising because their breasts had gotten smaller in size. Our genes determine certain physical characteristics such as the colour of our skin, hair, our height and even the breast size. There is no doubt that the breast size has various implications for a woman. Some base their sexuality and attractiveness on it. This is why we see a huge increase in breast implants and other procedures.

Suffice to say, it is more important to improve fitness levels and health than breast size.

Quick Facts

- Weight on the scale is a combination of fat, muscle, bones, organs, etc.
- Losing weight therefore is not always indicative of fat loss. You should aim to lose fat and build muscle.
- Losing weight with dieting alone, without the inclusion of exercise, will result in loss of muscle and some fat.
- The weighing scale, height/weight charts and BMI need to be kept in mind, and should not be the only guidelines by which to assess fitness.
- The measurement of the waist circumference using inch tape gives one a clear indication of fat loss in the abdomen, which not only has several health benefits, but is also cosmetically appealing.

- One can lose weight in various unsavoury ways. Point is, do they improve your health? Are they sustainable?
- Thin women seeking to gain weight should focus on weight training to build muscle and an appropriately increased, balanced, high nutritive food intake.

WHAT IS MORE IMPORTANT THAN JUST WEIGHT LOSS IS IMPROVED FITNESS LEVELS. Focus on the various aspects of your fitness, set appropriate goals and work towards improving fitness levels.

Questions & DIY

- What is your waist circumference?

- What is your waist hip ratio? Does it fall in the low risk category?

- Fill in the Body Statistics chart. Record values every month.

- Why are you exercising?

- If you are not, why not?

- What are the different ways you have tried to lose weight unsuccessfully in the past?
  1.
  2.
  3.
  4.

- How and why did you gain the weight again?

- How did it make you feel?

- What will you do different this time?

CHAPTER 2

THE BENEFITS OF FITNESS

GETTING FIT IS ABOUT MORE THAN JUST LOSING WEIGHT

What is the point in exercising or trying to get fit?

You may look at yourself and your life and say, 'Well, I am fine as I am, I may not be fit but what do I need to be fit for? I would rather eat whatever I want, relax, work if I can and just enjoy life.'

There is a saying that you cannot describe the view from the top of a hill to someone in the valley. It is hard to express exactly what it feels like to get and stay fit. One has to actually experience it.

Every woman needs a different impetus to begin exercise. For some it is plain vanity. They want to look great in a pair of jeans! For others it may be a health call, another may decide prevention is the way to go. You have to find your motivation.

> Tanya was a young woman who looked far younger than her 22 odd years. She didn't see any reason to exercise. She was underweight as far as I could see. Nonetheless, that was just the point. Young…

...women, who appear slim like Tanya, see no reason to sweat it out.

She had a family of people who did. Her father and her brother were fitness freaks, to put it in her own words. They had, as far as she could remember, tried to get her to start working out. Bullying, cajoling, threats...nothing worked. She saw absolutely no rationale in exercising.

One evening her mother came to me for fitness advice. Tanya came in with her, for want of something better to do. She was bright-eyed and bushy-tailed. I think curiosity got the better of her when she listened to the various ways in which one could approach fitness and the reasons why one should and could get fit. Perhaps, being intelligent and interested in a more holistic approach to fitness rather than the usual weight issue is what got her to join TFL.

She, herself, was the most surprised at her own enthusiasm about fitness. She loved it. Now she wants to be a fitness instructor, get certified and pursue it as a career option.

This makes me wonderfully happy, for I think we need more people who are passionate about holistic fitness, understand it deeply and truly want to make a difference.

Find your own incentive. Talk to people who exercise regularly. Talk to fitness freaks, as they are called, and professionals, so you may view exercise through a different lens.

> We can do nothing without the body, let us always take care that it is in its best condition to sustain us.
>
> —*Anon.*

You look better, you feel better, you are better.

I think most of us are quite familiar with the various benefits of fitness. They have been widely publicized, advertized, talked and written about all over the media. It makes for wonderful copy. Catchy clichés, like 'no pain, no gain', are solemn predictions of doomed health unless you exercise regularly. Clever ad campaigns by sports companies featuring stunningly beautiful athletes like Maria Sharapova or Sania Mirza are poignant reminders of the dreadful repercussions of a lazy lifestyle.

The power of advertising affects different people differently. I am reminded of an absolutely remarkable ad of an incredibly fit and good-looking man cycling up some treacherously steep path. He made it look exhilarating! This was so inspiring that I went rushing out and bought a bike the very next day and started biking as part of my fitness routine.

Of course, not everyone reacts like that. Alternately, other ad campaigns, which propagate the electrical ab-slimming belt for instance, have gullible consumers believe that they only have to strap the outrageous contraption around their waist and lie back in the luxury of their bed, maybe watch a mindless soap on TV, for that enviable waistline.

Most people, though, still manage to convince themselves that somehow all this hype about regular exercise does not apply to them. I see this predominantly among women who are not (yet) visibly overweight, but who may in fact be carrying around an inordinate amount of fat. Many obese women also choose to think that exercise is pointless.

At the other end of the spectrum are women who believe everything they read, obsess about their weight, fitness and bodies, starve themselves half to death, exercise till they drop and fantasize about looking like that super slim, Photoshopped and airbrushed creature on the cover of a glossy magazine.

Both kinds of women are at a risk of harming themselves. The former, because they can very easily slip from being slightly overweight to obese, with their fitness levels possibly sliding to an abysmal low without them even recognizing it. The latter could be more prone to eating disorders like anorexia and bulimia. They may abuse their bodies in the hope of being slim, read *beautiful*. They may even resort to some horrifying practices in the hope of losing weight.

BALANCE IS THE KEY TO WEIGHT AND HEALTH MANAGEMENT

Most people begin an exercise routine only when they absolutely HAVE to. A visit to their doctor has finally frightened them into believing that there is no other option but to fall in line and participate in this mundane, mindless business of fitness!

So, they drag themselves to a gym. Feel intimidated by the buff trainer, find fault with that terribly unnatural machine that makes one walk on a conveyor belt in the hope of losing weight, are horrified to see the strange-looking apparatus that supposedly strengthens their muscles, and slink away swearing they would much rather go for a more natural walk in the park or maybe do yoga.

Well, as long as one starts the ball rolling, there is some hope for progress towards a well-designed fitness routine.

Weight loss is one of the most common reasons people begin an exercise programme. However, exercise has a multitude of other benefits, weight loss and weight maintenance being only the tip of the iceberg. Going through the next few pages will help you understand the immense benefits of fitness. If this doesn't convince you, I am not sure what else will.

We have proven that it is cheaper and more effective to maintain good health than to regain it once it is lost.

—*Dr Kenneth Cooper, Father of Aerobics*

PHYSICAL BENEFITS OF EXERCISE

Vitamin X or exercise is the closest thing to an **anti-ageing pill** we will ever come across. None of the expensive anti-wrinkle or anti-ageing creams come close to a good 30-minute workout. Women (and men) spend hours in a beauty parlour trying to look better. The steady increase in the use of Botox, facelifts and tummy tucks indicates a society that is quite preoccupied with youth and beauty. How about 'healthy'? You could have it all, if you focus on getting your fitness act together. Well, within reason of course: running regularly will not turn you into a Shakira.

Mallika is a physician. She was dangerously overweight. She'd read the literature on obesity and its various health-related problems. For years, she dabbled in diets and some apology for exercise, didn't see results that were motivating enough, and fell off the wagon several times.

In 2008 she reached her nadir—her mother had passed away. It became evident to her that her mother's quality of life the last few years was appalling, because she had been grossly overweight and had suffered from every lifestyle disease conceivable. She decided to start working out.

By the time she came to meet me, she was already exercising regularly but had no idea what she was doing. She spent an hour every day in a gym, walked on the treadmill, pulled and pushed some weights, not quite sure how it helped.

She joined us in 2010 and started learning about the holistic concept of fitness and its various aspects (cardio, strength, flexibility, body composition, rest and nutrition). She is 50 years old but, being an avid learner, that didn't stop her from pursuing fitness with all the enthusiasm of a child.

She trains with weights twice a week, walks thrice a week, does aerobic classes twice a week and, besides her routine stretches, does yoga twice a week to sustain and improve her flexibility.

Her weight training is intense. Her cardio can now put a 25-year-old to shame.

She has to date lost 20 kg, lowered her fat percentage from 47 to 30 per cent and is quite literally on top of the world.

Sitting in her clinic one day, a family walked in for their appointment. They looked a bit concerned, whispered among themselves, and quickly left smiling apologetically. Mallika was confused—had she said or done something?

Outside, the father disclosed to the secretary, 'We came to see Dr Mallika, not her daughter; when will Dr Mallika be in?'

It took some convincing but finally the family was satisfied (and somewhat bemused) that this was the same woman, just a fabulously leaner, fitter version, who obviously looked 20 years younger. Mallika recalls this story at any given opportunity! Can you blame her?

Physical appearance: Certainly, a part of being successful is about external appearances. Being physically fit, with impeccable posture, improves the impression one creates, which, let's face it, is crucial in today's world. Furthermore, the results of engaging in a fitness routine are not just superficial, as they are, for instance, following plastic surgery, but internal as well, improving the condition of your muscles, bones, joints, blood vessels, even your brain, making you seem younger, preventing degeneration, which is otherwise inevitable.

The right kind of exercise will make you achieve a **slimmer, more toned**, sleeker silhouette. Clothes fit better, and you walk tall with improved posture.

Along with your calcium and vitamin B complex, I suggest you make vitamin X a non-negotiable part of your day.

Improved posture: Posture is a combination of proper muscle strength, balance, alignment, body awareness and an inner confidence. If the muscles of the upper back, shoulders, abdomen and core are weak, the natural tendency is to slouch forward and assume the most comfortable posture—that of a slob! The impression you communicate is one lacking in confidence, and it could cost you some opportunities in career and relationships. Working on your muscles to increase strength and balance, is the first step towards improving posture.

The cerebral work, of course, remains. Although one can mimic confidence with great posture, it helps if one can actually develop it from within as well! Ironically, exercising regularly improves self-confidence from within!

Improved energy levels: Improving your stamina or cardiovascular endurance will not only help you perform your workout better and more easily, but will translate into real-life situations as well. The loss of weight and the participation in an exercise programme increase energy levels contrary to the common belief that exercise will tire you. Sometimes when you are feeling a slump in your energy levels, instead of reaching for a cup of java, try a quick brisk walk, even within the office or home, up and down the corridors and stairs. You will find it perks you up.

Being overweight can be downright exhausting. What with having to haul all that extra weight around all day, feeling your knees and back hurt when you climb stairs, God help you if you have to, feeling irritable at having to wait in queues, annoyed at having to carry grocery bags as your man or woman Friday is not around, or wanting to lie down after attempting any kind of housework...You can't seem to be able to do anything without taking a break! Your couch is your only friend.

Weight loss: Of course regular exercise will help you lose fat, when done correctly and balanced with your diet. I have deliberately not listed this benefit of exercise at the top of the list because it is not the only one you should obsess about. Weight is a reference point that you should keep in mind.

You get stronger: I can just hear you say, why would I need to be strong? I have a husband or boyfriend to lift my bags (yeah right!), maids to do the physical labour at home, etc.

This is the twenty-first century, ladies. Strong is in! Even if only to lift your LV bags off the conveyor belt at the airport.

There is a certain confidence and pride that comes with being able to handle physical work on your own without having to whine to a male counterpart even about opening a pickle bottle for you. You can be sure that you can manage the housework if your maid plays truant. You can carry your kid and a grocery bag if so required, carry your laptop on your shoulder without ending up with a pain in the neck, walk up and down the stairs. All these are simple daily chores that one sometimes takes for granted. A client once told me how she used to, for the longest time, only negotiate stairs gingerly by holding the railing and placing both feet on each and every step. After beginning training with weights to strengthen her lower body, losing weight and improving her balance, now she says she literally bounds up and down the staircase.

PSYCHOLOGICAL AND EMOTIONAL BENEFITS

Exercise boosts your mood: The release of endorphins in the brain with increased physical activity makes you feel good. This feel-good factor often lasts all day, keeping you in a positive frame of mind. In addition to looking better, one feels better. It's no wonder then that regular exercisers come back day after day for their fix. Once accustomed to that incredible feeling, it is hard to go through a day without it. I have had clients tell me they make better spouses, daughters and mothers after beginning to exercise. Exercise is addictive!

> At a social gathering, as I stood chatting with some women, I felt a tug at my sari. Turning around I saw the most adorable 8-year-old, with big glasses and a million-dollar smile that exposed two missing teeth.
>
> 'You know my mummy,' she said. 'When is she going to come back to exercise again?' We had cancelled classes for a month for various reasons and intended to resume in a couple of days, 'She must! She is so much more fun and plays with me when she goes to her class every day.' Right out of the mouth of a babe!

Stress relief and protection against the harmful effects of too much stress: Modalities like yoga and t'ai chi come under the realm of mind–body exercises that focus specifically on the breath and the connection between the breath and the body. In these, the conscious breathing, the slow nature of the exercise-form and introspection create a meditative experience.

I believe, however, that **any form of exercise can be meditative if you want it to be.** All forms have a mind–body connection. There is no closer demonstration of this mind–body connection than a marathon runner completing her run, for instance. Without your mind you can hardly get in a good workout of any sort.

> Sandra is a mother of three young children. Her life revolves around getting them organized, fed and taken care of. Her husband travels extensively, so most of the time she has to manage home and kids on her own. Sometimes it can be overwhelming.
>
> Without her fitness routine every evening before the kids...

...come home, she says, she would probably be a wreck. Her routine keeps her grounded:

- She runs 3.7 miles 4 times a week,
- does yoga twice a week,
- and weight-trains twice a week.

The one hour that she spends by herself, revelling in her solitude and focusing on her own body, prepares her to be a caregiver to her children when she has to. I love her focus and dedication to herself. That is just the thing that makes her a great mother as well.

The repetitive, rhythmic muscular action of the exercise diverts the mind from the stress factor to the action at hand, relieving stressful energy. This gradually reduces the levels of the stress hormone cortisol and increases endorphins, which in turn makes one feel better. Physical activity also appears to provide some amount of immunity toward future stress, meaning that those who exercise regularly seem to be able to handle stress better and have a better physiological response to stress.

More self-confidence: An increase in self-confidence arises out of one's own body awareness and the realization of one's capabilities. Being able to exercise regularly and lose weight is not a simple or easy undertaking. When it is achieved, there is a sense of accomplishment.

The simple key is the focus that physical exercise demands. This is when total attention is on one's self and one's physical being, even if only for about an hour. This diversion seems somehow necessary for us to balance out the rest of the day, which is frenzied with activity, mundane, stressful or exhilarating, usually involving other people. It is almost as if one confers meditatively with oneself in this physical act that requires the use of one's body.

Spending such quality time with oneself does wonders for your self-confidence. I have seen women blossom and become different people after they start and manage to stick with an exercise programme. How could just doing something simple like walking every day allow people to improve their self-confidence, you ask? Well it just does. The endorphins in their brain have something to do with their cheerier behaviour for sure, but it's also about them achieving something significant like weight loss, looking better, basking in the compliments and attention, which apparently improve their personalities.

'Of course I am more confident now. Knocking off all that fat was not easy AT ALL. But now I feel I can do anything.' Sameera is a high-powered executive. She was at the top of her game career-wise. Yet, there were reservations about her true capability. She believed deep down that she did not 'truly have it in her to do what it takes.' Her several failed attempts at weight loss over the years had depleted her confidence.

Her problem was simple: she wanted the easy way out. Anything for a quick fix. Initially she just could not get past the fact that I insisted that fitness was a lifelong plan not some short-term remedy.

'But I only want to lose 8 kg,' was her constant plea.

'And then what?' I asked her.

'What do you mean, then what?'

'I mean, and then what happens? You stop exercising, forget to eat healthy, grow older and gain all that weight, and more, yet again?'

'Isn't there any way I can lose weight and keep it off?' She was unconvinced.

'Of course, keep training.' She looked at me balefully.

After several sessions with her, she committed to a fitness programme for 6 months. Over the course of those months, her progress was not straightforward. Her constant battle with a...

...need for a timeline after which she could stop exercising prevented her from really applying herself.

Another problem was her obsession with the scale. She was literally in a panic on the day of the reassessment. 'What if I haven't lost weight? I will be so depressed!' she declared. She had already signed her treaty with depression.

I was slowly losing patience explaining the facts about weight on the scale not being the only indicator of size, and so on. In reality, there had been a remarkable difference physically. Her waist measurement had dropped 5 cm, and her cardiovascular endurance and strength improved remarkably. Fortunately, her scale also showed a drop in weight.

Three more months and she had lost more weight. I could see that she was calmer and seemed inclined to take exercise more seriously and not just as a means to weight loss alone.

After 6 months, she was on top of the world. I told her she had lost 5 per cent fat. She was a little sceptical about the value of fat percentage, but more thrilled about the new shape she had acquired. Her confidence was soaring.

I worry. She has to be off on a long sojourn abroad. She promises to train regularly, And declares she will 'join a gym, run, do yoga, anything you say.'

She keeps in touch on email and Skype. She seems to be doing well. She fills in her food and exercise journal, which has become her bible. She says, it keeps her motivated. She can't wait to get back to learn a new routine.

MEDICAL BENEFITS

If we could give every individual the right amount of nourishment and exercise, not too little and not too much, we would have found the safest way to health.

—*Hippocrates*

Another benefit of weight loss is simply a better **quality of life**, wherein your risk to disease is reduced. A family history of diabetes does increase your risk to the disease statistically, but the disease is not unavoidable. **A healthy lifestyle of exercise and diet can keep diabetes at bay, and if already evident can at least be managed better.**

Regular participation in any aerobic activity will improve the condition of your heart and lungs—the cardiorespiratory system—keeping it fit and protecting it from coronary heart disease.

Several studies have shown that some very common ailments that afflict human beings today can be managed quite effectively with regular exercise that is well structured to suit the individual.

Research has found that several medical problems can be effectively managed with exercise:

- **Obesity:** Yes, this is considered a disease! Exercise and diet is the mainstay of treatment to assist weight loss. Loss of fat can improve quality of life.
- **Diabetes mellitus (Type 2)** is primarily lifestyle-related. Managing the disease, and even preventing it, is possible with exercise and diet. In a pre–diabetic, exercise prevented progression to frank diabetes by 58 per cent.
- **Heart disease** can occur as a result of high cholesterol, diabetes, obesity, and so on. The incidence of heart disease increases primarily because of unhealthy lifestyle habits including sedentary living and poor diet. Managing these aspects of your lifestyle goes a long way in keeping your heart healthy.
- **Metabolic syndrome** is a combination of abdominal obesity, abnormal sugar and elevated cholesterol levels. It is more prevalent now, and Indian men and women seem

to be more prone to it. A sedentary lifestyle supplemented with rich, calorie-laden food makes it very easy to develop this condition.

- **Hypothyroidism:** Weight gain is common with hypothyroidism. Losing it is possible with the right medication and exercise.

- **Polycystic ovaries** are diagnosed in many young women today. It is a cause of great heartache, especially when it leads to difficulty in conceiving. Regular physical exercise has seen improved fertility rates besides weight loss and regularized cycles.

- **Menopausal symptoms** drive many women crazy. Exercise is beneficial in managing symptoms like mood swings and weight gain. Hot flushes, however, are often not managed with exercise alone.

- **Osteoporosis** or fragile bones leading to fractures, especially in older women, can be prevented with weight training. Postmenopausal women had a 41 per cent reduction in risk of hip fracture with just 4 hours of exercise per week.

- **Fibromyalgia** or generalized body pain and trigger-point pain, is often associated with fatigue and depression. Moderate intensity aerobic activity will improve overall well-being and physical functionality.

- **Hypertension and stroke:** High blood pressure is very often the cause of a stroke. Management of elevated blood pressure with exercise, diet and weight loss has been researched and established.

- **Back pain due to poor posture** can be the result of a weak core or back muscles, and abdominal obesity. Back pain is almost a universal complaint of women over the age of 40. Shockingly, I find even young women in their thirties suffer incapacitating back pain that brings them to a physician. Proper muscle strengthening and stretching can both prevent and treat most of these women.

- **High cholesterol levels** due to poor diet, lack of exercise and obesity can cause heart disease. Effective lifestyle management with exercise and diet is critical in the treatment of this problem.

- **Knee arthritis:** One hour of exercise will reduce pain and disability by 47 per cent. Weight-training to strengthen the muscles around the knee, stretching to maintain flexibility of lower legs and weight maintenance are the key to managing symptoms of arthritis.

- **Reduced progression to Alzheimer's and dementia by 50 per cent:** Exercise helps with improved blood circulation to the brain, and improved cognition and memory in the prevention of these disorders.

- **Anxiety:** Symptoms of anxiety can be reduced with therapeutic exercise by about 48 per cent. Breathing, yoga and meditation have been found to be effective.

- **Depression** symptoms are elevated by almost 47 per cent with regular exercise, which has been found to be as effective as antidepressants in some studies. It is definitely a mainstay of supplementary treatment for depression. **A low mood** is improved with just 20 minutes of physical exercise.

- **Premenstrual symptoms:** Some women suffer from extreme symptoms during their premenstrual period. Even moderate intensity exercise seems to alleviate symptoms. It is a myth that you cannot exercise during your periods. You may not be able to do as much, but do something. It keeps you feeling positive, and reduces the pain to a large extent.

BEING SEDENTARY IS BAD FOR HEALTH!

A study done in Australia by Dr Lennert Veerman of the School of Population Health at the University of Queensland reported, in the *British Journal of Sports Medicine*, that watching an average of 2 hours of TV a day could reduce life expectancy by 1.8 years for men and 1.5 years for women! A similar finding of reduced life expectancy was found in the year 2010 by Prof. David Dunstan. His team estimated that every hour of TV watched after the age 25 is associated with a reduction in life expectancy of 22 minutes.

A study in *The Lancet* finds that even 15 minutes of exercise can reduce a person's risk of death by 14 per cent. This is encouraging for people who find it hard to exercise continuously for the recommended 30 minutes at a time.

> Walking is man's best medicine.
> —*Hippocrates*

I must mention here that although exercise is not a panacea for all the ailments of modern society, it is definitely an easily accessible, highly affordable and simple form of preventive care.

ECONOMIC BENEFITS

> Physical fitness is not only one of the most important keys to a healthy body; it is the basis of dynamic and creative intellectual activity.
> —*John F. Kennedy*

A healthy workforce is crucial for the economy of any organization. Regular exercise improves memory, acumen and alertness, all critical in the working environment. **Top-level managers who exercise are better decision makers.**

Employees who exercise regularly are more productive, taking fewer days of sick leave making them assets and not liabilities to the company. Research done in several corporate organizations shows that the inclusion of fitness has benefitted employees, increasing efficiency.

On an individual level, **being fit has several economic benefits, one of the most obvious being the reduced cost of medical bills!** Not having long-term, degenerative diseases frees up one's finances to do other things in life. Hospital stay, surgery, medication, nursing care, physiotherapy, all of which cost a lot of money, can be avoided. The financial and emotional expense of ill health is often grossly underestimated. This could be kept to the minimum by just incorporating a few sensible lifestyle choices.

Over the years I have spoken to several groups of corporate women from various organizations. Some of these organizations have their own fitness facilities within the premises, which are

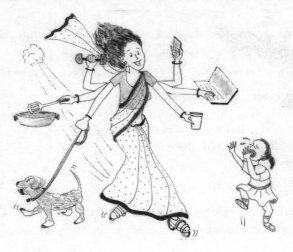

rarely used by the women, I am told. They have to rush home to cook for the children and husband; they cannot waste time in a gym. And yet, there are several of them being diagnosed with diabetes, hypertension, and so on, every day.

They are happy to have regular health check-ups organized by the company, though. They get their blood pressure, blood sugar and haemoglobin checked, they are told what medication to take, and continue with their lives without considering that perhaps they could be more proactive with their own health instead of being mere witnesses to a script being played out. I find this attitude, especially among working women, particularly agonizing. These women take responsibility for their families and contribute greatly to their financial maintenance and yet are unable to set aside some time for themselves to improve their own health and well-being.

Here's the reality—the fitter you are, the more you are able to do without tiring easily. You are in a better frame of mind to deal with a crisis, you don't have your own aches and pains to contend with, you are more agile, sharp and energized. You don't feel depressed or irritable. You achieve more in the day than you ever thought possible!

IMPROVED QUALITY OF LIFE

Being fit, opens up a completely new world of opportunities for recreational activity that life has to offer. A holiday could now mean physical activity without tiring; playing with the kids or pets is not an exhausting chore or something you try to avoid any more. Housework doesn't half kill you. Suffice to say that one of the greatest benefits of a fitness programme is just simply a **better quality of life**. It is an ongoing process, where you learn something about yourself every day. If you are patient and persistent, the rewards are well worth the effort.

CHAPTER 3

WOMEN AND FITNESS

OUR UNIQUE APPROACH TO FITNESS

There's no easy way out. If there was, I would have bought it, and
believe me, it would have been one of my favorite things.

—*Oprah Winfrey on exercise*

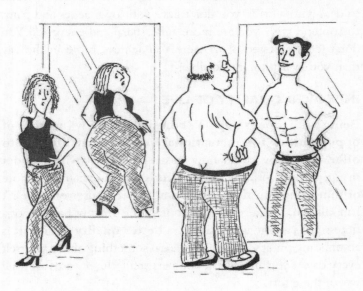

Some of us are so self-depreciative. So easily disheartened by the false, overly critical image we have of ourselves. We do not need to turn into pure narcissists, but it would help us all immensely if only we were a little kinder to ourselves. Instead of working against the body we so obviously hate, we could work with it, creating a more nurturing environment to improve fitness, lose weight, etc.

We have to understand that there are several differences between men and women, besides the obvious of course! In fact, a lot of recent research focuses on **gender-specific medicine**. Women's bodies respond differently to exercise and food. Men on average have a higher muscle mass and therefore a higher metabolic rate. They tend to lose fat faster if they make even small changes in their diet and exercise just a little harder. Women, on the other hand, usually find it harder to lose fat. This can be disastrous as when a couple resolves to lose weight together, the man invariably loses it faster.

Nitya and her fiancé, Rajiv, decided to get on a fitness programme together. When they met me, she was already exercising, and training with weights. He was more laid-back. His attitude was, 'Just tell me what to do, and I will do it.'

She was always negotiating, 'But can I eat chocolate just once a day? Can I eat out at least twice a week? Can I skip my cardio today and do more tomorrow?'

A month down the road. He had lost 5 kg, increased tremendously in strength and was running easily on the treadmill at 6-8 mph. Nitya had lost 2 kg. The other aspects of her fitness had definitely improved, but she was irate at not having lost as much weight as Rajiv!

I pointed out that she had a negative attitude towards her body. She was barely overweight but was constantly pinching the little fat around her tummy and moaning! Rajiv, on the other...

...hand, came into the gym, worked out, gave it his best, and left without being too concerned about timelines or the weighing scale and was rarely critical about his appearance! He enjoyed his workout, laughed, teased her, decided he would train to run a marathon and focused primarily on that rather than his weight.

'This is not a competition between the two of you,' I warned Nitya. 'For your own sake, I suggest you make it your own journey, not a contest. Focus on what you have achieved not what you haven't achieved in comparison to him.'

Having worked with **Indian women** for close to two decades, I have had the pleasure and privilege of seeing their different avatars. Their strength, vulnerability, versatility, reticence, resilience, pain, joy, martyrdom, and so much more... Indian women have a struggle slightly different from their Western counterparts. They have family, extended family, in-laws, outlaws, societal pressures, and a lot more than they can sometimes deal with. Many middle-class women are now dominant breadwinners for their family. They commute, earn, play the power game with the men, take care of the children and husband, cook and clean, are responsible for their parents and in-laws, make enormous, critical financial and family decisions, and are the fulcrum of the family and society. Keeping in good health then becomes even more important.

However, there are some of us who are completely delusional about our health and fitness, appearance, shape and size.

- We are obese and believe we are just slightly overweight, or pleasantly plump.
- We endure an excruciating existence with back pain and discomfort, but tell ourselves that it is in our genes and therefore we cannot help what we look like; we endure

poor fitness levels and weight gain telling ourselves, that's how it is in our family, and so on.

BEGIN WITH APPRECIATING YOUR BODY THE WAY IT IS

The first step into a fitness routine is to accept and love your body the way it is. You have done this to yourself over the years—neglect, self-abuse perhaps, a flippant attitude about food and health. Whatever the cause, you have achieved it single-handedly, maybe with a little help from the chaatwala or the gourmet chocolate store down the street. The important thing therefore is to appreciate that despite all the neglect and abuse, your body is still serving you, protesting often, but still struggling to keep pace with your debauchery.

If you suffer from stress, anxiety, depression, hypothyroidism or other medical disorders that could be contributing to, but are not the undisputed cause of, your weight woes, they need to be addressed accordingly. Many hormonal imbalances and mood disorders can make fat loss more difficult, but not impossible. It just requires a slightly different and more composite, holistic approach with the inclusion of any one or all of the following:

- Relaxation techniques
- Breathing routines that can be done every day and have been shown to help lower stress levels.
- Meditation
- Cognitive behavioural therapy or CBT, which is the retraining of the mind to change its thought process to a more beneficial and positive approach.

'I am being treated for an anxiety disorder,' Amitha announced on my first consultation with her. 'I have been told I will find it very difficult to lose weight because I suffer from stress and anxiety.'

Amitha, like many young women today, multitasks between being supermom and successful career woman. Her job takes her to various parts of the world. She travels at least once a month. Add to that the deadlines, school plays and play dates, running a home with two young children and a husband who is also almost married to his job (her theory)—she had her hands full. It was no wonder she was stressed and suffered an anxiety disorder. She needed pills to sleep, she was on antidepressants and extremely overweight.

'If that is what you believe, why have you come to me?' I asked.

'I wanted someone to help me with it.' I was a bit confused, but she carried on, 'If you can get me to lose weight I think I would feel better about myself and have more energy.'

'How do you think I am going to do that?' I asked.

'Well I don't know, but I have been told that I won't be able to lose weight because of my anxiety and stress. I am borderline diabetic and my cholesterol is high, so I really don't know what to do.'

We were in a quandary. As was obvious, Amitha had already decided she could not lose weight and that the cause of her weight was her stress and anxiety.

This needed more than just walking on a treadmill and some push-ups.

I had her see my psychologist to start cognitive behavioural therapy as part of her weight loss programme. She was only too happy to start CBT, as to her, anxiety was the root cause of all evil.

Over the next 6 months she had to come to terms with some facts:
- Although she did lead a highly stressful life, she did not have to be a victim of her circumstances all the time.
- She did have a choice with all the decisions that she made, provided she was willing to face the consequences.

- Anxiety was indeed a disease, but the kind that required patient participation in its management.
- Changing one's thought process by reconditioning the mind takes time but is not impossible, and this could be the key to being able to treat anxiety and depression.
- Travel abroad did not necessarily mean she could not exercise. In fact, the beautiful hotels she stayed in gave her access to the best gyms and swimming pools. (She did use hotel facilities, except, she only headed for the sauna with the hope of losing weight!)
- If she believed her children were her priority, as she claimed, she would need to make some compromises with work. Her main bone of contention, it appeared, was that her husband didn't pull his weight at home! She had to be taught that we were now focusing on her and her ability to manage her stress properly, not compound it by expecting others to fall in line.
- Regular exercise would definitely help her stay fit and lose fat irrespective of her disease, provided she was willing to accept responsibility for certain behavioural patterns such as her erratic diet.

She had a lot of work to do. She had reached a point where she was ready to do so. Her fitness is ongoing and she is showing remarkable results.

When you begin your journey into fitness with respect for your body, and treat it with the dignity it deserves, it will respond better to what you are asking of it.

I see, instead, women who come in with standard statements like 'I hate my body,' 'I hate my fat thighs.' Well, there you go, you have begun communicating with your body on the wrong foot already. All the negativity, stress, anger, shame and disgust towards yourself and your body, does not help the weight loss process.

Have you noticed that ever so often a new fitness fad comes

along and everyone attempts to be a part of it? It could be tae-bo, Zumba, kick-boxing or belly dancing. They are all variations of cardio activities to break the monotony of and add some excitement and novelty to your fitness routine.

The proponents of the given fitness form will have you believe it is the ultimate phenomenon that ever benefitted mankind, that it will result in the best body you can ever dream of. Clever marketing will even lead you to believe you could be that girl in the TV ad with the flat stomach and skimpy clothes gyrating effortlessly to some exotic rhythm. Yes, it may be good for her, she may enjoy it, stick with it, be good at it, and so on; but does it work for you? The form of exercise you follow needs to be determined by you and you alone. Understanding where it fits into your fitness routine and what else you need to incorporate to achieve holistic health are questions that you should consider.

Once they achieve a certain level of fitness, I usually encourage women to cross-train or try different cardio activities. This serves two purposes; it challenges the body to respond better and differently, get fitter and lose those last few kilos. More importantly, it prevents boredom.

This is a question I get all the time: 'If I stop exercising, will I gain weight?'

Here are two simple equations:

1. You exercise $\Rightarrow$ you burn calories $\Rightarrow$ your calorie intake is less than expenditure $\Rightarrow$ you lose fat

2. You stop exercising $\Rightarrow$ you do not burn those extra calories $\Rightarrow$ if your calorie intake remains the same as when you were exercising $\Rightarrow$ you gain fat

'Doctor, I don't want to start exercising,' Anya declared. 'How else can you get me to lose weight?'

'If you only want to lose weight, why don't you starve yourself?' She didn't miss the sarcasm.

'You know I can't do that, it's not good for health.'

'Okay, so let me get this straight, why don't you want to start exercising?' I already knew the answer, but I asked anyway.

'Because I have done it before and when I stopped, I gained all the weight back! I can't let that happen again!'

'So why did you stop?'

'How can I keep doing it?' she was incredulous. 'You expect me to keep exercising even after I lose weight?'

'Well, yes, that's the general idea. You know exercise has several other benefits, Anya, why are you focused on the weight? If you continue to exercise—you get to keep the weight off AND enjoy the other benefits. Isn't that a good enough reason?'

'I don't know, Doctor! They say you feel better and all that stuff. But I feel good anyway, so why torture myself?' I could not help laughing. She had a point. She was a very positive and infectiously cheerful person.

'So how about we make a deal. I will try not to make it torturous and you try to stick with it. I can tell you one thing for sure, if you do go on a starvation diet to lose weight you certainly will not keep feeling as good as you do now. By the way, how many diets have you followed to date?'

'Let's see, Atkins, South Beach, North Beach, General Motors, Paleo, Kellogg's Special K...I have lost count. The weight always comes back.'

'So here's a fascinating fact, you do invariably need to go off a difficult diet because it is not sustainable. However, you really do not need to go off exercise and balanced eating. This is about learning to eat the right way, not go on a diet as you see it. It is also learning to actually enjoy exercise. That way it becomes sustainable.'

'You are kidding, right? Enjoy exercise? That's like saying you can actually learn to enjoy holding your breath!'

And so it went on. She finally succumbed to the idea of working out. She would grumble about it every day. My trainers were very good with her. I told her she needed to grow up and be mature about not wanting to be entertained by her workout all the time. She had to 'Just Do It'.

She still has a shaky relationship with fitness. Deep down she knows there is no other way, but I find she is often kicking and screaming her way into the gym. There are many women like her. They just never get to accept or even like exercise.

But. I still have hope for Anya...

IS ENGAGING IN FITNESS A FRIVOLOUS ACTIVITY?

It may appear so when you consider the enormous responsibility that a woman encounters in the prime of her life. **Where is the time for exercise?**

The **reproductive years** leave very little time for oneself. The children are growing up and require your attention. You are busy making your way through your career while also managing home. Your husband is probably coping with his own work crisis. It may appear difficult to set aside time for something as seemingly frivolous as fitness.

Look at It This Way...

You have a huge number of responsibilities; you need to be at the top of your game. You need to be in good health, stay fit, positive and energetic. If something as simple as an hour exercising can help you achieve all of this, would it not be worth allocating time for it?

View it as an hour you spend engaging in an activity that is improving you on the inside—heart, lungs, muscles, tendons, bones, mood, self-esteem—and the outside—your appearance, skin, posture, muscle tone and shape. Consider, too, that this hour you spend on yourself will improve your ability to deal with the rest of your day.

- It will put you in a better frame of mind to address domestic and professional challenges.
- Keep you energized throughout the day to multitask.
- Keep you looking good so you feel good, more confident and attractive.

SOME OBSERVATIONS PERTAINING TO WOMEN AND FITNESS

However much they require it, only a certain segment of women come forward to join a fitness routine, or at least attempt to. It is either the younger women, possibly unmarried, or going to be married, who have the motivation to lose weight; or the older women, whose children have left home and who have already developed various lifestyle diseases like diabetes, hypertension, etc. **The women in between are too busy just getting on with life.**

The busier the women, the more likely they are to somehow find the time to work out. Perhaps busy, productive women know how to manage their time better. They also value their time more and so eliminate the 'time wasters' as far as possible.

Others find a zillion excuses:

- The husband needs me, I have to cook for him. *While he is in the gym getting a good workout.*
- Facebook needs me.
- The children need me.
- My boss needs me.
- I have to work.
- I have an assignment.
- I have to travel.
- I have guests.
- I have an important TV programme.

- I am really not that fat, I don't think I need to exercise. *Did I mention exercise was not just about weight loss?*
- I have to cook and clean. *All day?*
- I have a card party where I have to sit on my butt and play a card game all evening.
- It's raining. *The aerobic class is indoors!*
- It's too hot. *The gym is air-conditioned!*
- My husband likes me overweight. *Really?*
- I am slim. *By what standards? Height and weight charts are to be kept in perspective. Body composition is more important.*

The list is endless. In fact, I am always surprised at the innovative excuses! Unfortunately, none of them are good enough.

Time Wasters You Can Do Without

- An unhealthy addiction to every possible TV serial.
- Mindless web-surfing. The internet can be a blessing and a curse, depending on how you use it.
- Playing online games all the time.
- Telephone conversations and emails that can be postponed to another day when you **do** have the time to waste—obviously there are some mails and some calls you need to attend to ASAP, others can wait for an appropriate time.
- Lack of planning, organization and prioritization can lead to a lot of time wasted on a job that could be accomplished quickly.
- Unwanted interruptions from friends and colleagues leading to meandering conversations.
- Long-winding meetings that seem not to accomplish anything in particular.
- Social meetings that never end and could be scheduled for another time when you can afford to socialize.
- Relatives dropping in unannounced, expecting to be entertained.

- Too many people who use you as a sounding board or a shoulder to cry on resulting in you never having some quality time for yourself.
- Am sure you can name many more.

ONCE A LIFESTYLE DISEASE IS ESTABLISHED

The consequences you face later in life for not taking care of your body, like weight gain, high cholesterol levels, diabetes and back pain, are a result of your own life choices, negligence, laziness and the lack of prioritization. These conditions are called lifestyle diseases, as they are mostly a consequence of poor lifestyle habits.

Once any of these problems are diagnosed, however, you can still be proactive in the management of the disease. Your role in the treatment of such diseases is crucial. Instead of leaving the success of treatment to doctors, divine intervention or pure quackery, get practical and take things into your own hands. Learn how to manage the disease and what you can do to contribute to your own well-being. Most of these problems require you to be more active, start exercising, and include stress management techniques. Your doctor can only prescribe medication, advise exercise, surgery, and so on. The actual execution is **your** responsibility.

You may need to make some adjustments to fit yourself in a regular fitness routine initially. Perhaps waking up half an hour earlier or missing a TV serial, *trust me, you'll survive it*, but as you get accustomed to it and start seeing positive results, you'll see that these are not compromises at all. Your confidence will grow along with your strength and stamina.

You will never look back.

Many of us stand in our own way, tripping ourselves up

with our numerous excuses, self-pity and delusions, preventing our own progress. We tend to set up roadblocks for ourselves and then say, 'I can't do it, there are too many hurdles.'

Questions & DIY

- Do you exercise every day? Yes/No
- Do you think you should? Yes/No
  If yes, why?

  If no, why?

- Have you started an exercise programme before and stopped? Yes/No
  If yes, why?

- What do you want to do different this time?

- By exercise what exactly do you mean?

CHAPTER 4

THE 4 PILLARS OF FITNESS
THE BASIC FOUNDATION OF FITNESS

Now that it is established **that weight is not the only measure of fitness**, let us take a peek at what really is.

It takes more than a certain number on the scale to qualify you as being fit. It does you no good to have a slim body with cholesterol levels that are way above normal. Neither is it acceptable to look great but have abnormal blood sugar, high blood pressure, depression, or other lifestyle diseases. What would be the point of being able to fit into a certain size jeans if you have appalling posture or backache that is near killing you?

When you consider being fit, you need to look at your body from a broader perspective, not only its **size and shape**. The internal workings of the human body are just as important as looking great.

- Having normal blood sugar and cholesterol levels.
- Maintaining a normal blood pressure.
- Being emotionally and physically stable.
- Being able to lead a good quality life.

- Being able to function productively through the day, both at work and at home.
- Remaining independent for as long as possible.
- Finally, also being able to enjoy life's recreational activities without falling apart.

Participating in a fitness routine will benefit anyone. The prescribed schedule should be comparable to a doctor's prescription in that it has to be individualized for that specific woman. It has to take into account her age, lifestyle, goals, current health status and fitness levels, body type, diet, travel, work environment and the various other aspects that make her needs unique. This prescription also changes with age and life situations.

The following are the **4 major pillars of fitness**, not necessarily in order of importance. The significance of each pillar and the time spent developing it will depend once again on individual goals and requirements.

1. **Stamina** is the measure of the fitness level of your heart and lungs and how efficiently they supply the working muscles with oxygen to work. Walking, running, cycling or spinning, swimming, aerobic dance, stepper, kick-boxing, etc. will improve stamina.

2. **Strength** is the measure of the strength of your muscles, or their ability to contract and work against resistance. Weight training, own-body weight resistance training, ashtanga yoga and other modalities that involve working the muscles against resistance will improve strength.

3. **Muscle endurance** is the ability of the muscle to work for a long duration of time without fatigue.

4. **Flexibility** is the measure of how supple each of your muscles or groups of muscles are. Simple stretches or hatha yoga will help improve flexibility.

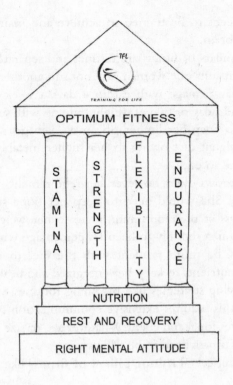

OPTIMUM FITNESS

STAMINA

STRENGTH

FLEXIBILITY

ENDURANCE

NUTRITION

REST AND RECOVERY

RIGHT MENTAL ATTITUDE

GET SIZE WISE

To have the best shape, size and fitness level you possibly can and stay that way, you need:

- **The 4 pillars:** Stamina, strength, endurance and flexibility.
- **Nutrition:** Obtaining a deep understanding of food groups and serving sizes, and balancing your diet so you can eat for optimum health, fitness and body fat.
- **Rest and recovery:** Achieving balance between training the body and resting it, for the most favourable results.
- **Attitude is everything!** The most important muscle

that needs to be trained to achieve and maintain fitness is the brain.

The 4 pillars of fitness are distinct and separate from each other. What suits one woman may not suit another. A younger woman may manage with cardio 4 days a week to improve stamina and a day or two of weight training with some cursory stretches to keep her limber. She may even get away with a more indulgent diet owing to her higher metabolism, active lifestyle, and so on.

As she grows older, however, her requirements will change perceptibly. She would need to keep her bone strength and muscle mass at their optimum, increase her weight training, address stamina sensibly to keep fat percentage within normal parameters, be more prudent with the diet to include the necessary nutrients to keep her energized and healthy, include stress-relieving strategies like breathing routines, yoga, and so on. All of this requires extensive communication between the fitness professional and client. Whatever age or size you are, the 4 pillars of fitness need to be addressed.

There are several **minor pillars of fitness** like:

- Speed
- Power
- Agility
- Reaction time
- Reflexes
- Coordination

Many of these need to be specifically addressed for athletes and sports persons depending on their sport. For a recreational fitness enthusiast, however, once the 4 Major Pillars are addressed, one can gradually focus on other important aspects of fitness, such as balance and core strength for the older woman.

For instance, in an unfit 80-year-old woman, the development of balance, strength and flexibility is more important than getting her to run a marathon. Although there *are* many 70-plus women running and even winning marathons, you won't hear of too many in that league. Most 70-plus women unfortunately have already thrown in the towel, given in to their ailments and lead a retired life. My 75-year-old mother is probably one of the few women I know personally who at her age is still terribly focused on her walking, weight training and yoga.

On the other hand, **engaging in a particular form of fitness activity in order to develop a certain pillar of fitness can also advance other aspects of fitness.** For example, a step class to improve stamina will also develop your coordination, reflexes and memory, as you try to remember choreography and music. It is quite amazing how the human body responds to physical and mental stimuli.

Many of my students, who came in as novices with two left feet and a great deal of apprehension, are now thoroughly enjoying complicated aerobic routines. This is one of the great benefits of group classes. The very nature of the class encourages you to engage in various aspects of fitness including your social skills!

My sincere advice, however, is **to build a strong foundation for your fitness by initially participating in simple options like walking for stamina, weight training for strength, and simple stretches for flexibility, and then move on to other forms and combinations of exercises.**

Learn to walk before you run. Strengthen your muscles, particularly your core muscles, before experimenting with complex moves. You don't want to injure your back gyrating with poor core strength in a Zumba class, or injure your knees stepping up and down with poor strength in your thigh muscles in a step class. This is why strength training that is specific and directed towards individual muscles is crucial in preventing injury. A strong body will also enable you to enjoy a variety of different types of fitness classes.

Questions & DIY

- Name the 4 pillars of fitness:
  1-
  2-
  3-
  4-
- Name 3 options to improve each of them:
  1-
  2-
  3-
- How do you aim to achieve optimum fitness?

CHAPTER 5

PILLAR I

STAMINA OR CARDIOVASCULAR ENDURANCE

> If it weren't for the fact that the TV set and the refrigerator are so
> far apart, some of us wouldn't get any exercise at all.
>
> —*Joey Adams*

How do you improve your stamina? By engaging what we affectionately call cardio. Any activity that keeps your heart rate elevated and keeps you breathing with some effort is referred to as aerobics, and will improve your stamina.

A SHORT HISTORY OF AEROBICS

Aerobic means 'with oxygen'. When the working muscles have a constant supply of oxygen to function, they are said to work aerobically. When the oxygen supply runs out or the body is unable to keep up with the demand, for instance when you perform sudden bursts of very intense exercise like sprinting, or lifting a very heavy weight, the muscles work **anaerobically**.

Any steady-state, moderate-paced workout is aerobic in nature. You are burning calories with the continuous motion.

Over time, however, your body adapts to this level of intensity and requires challenge.

In the path-breaking book *Aerobics*, Dr Kenneth Cooper elucidates the benefits of regular aerobic activity. He emphasizes the need for increasing aerobic activity by increasing the **number of steps walked per day to 10,000.** Dr Cooper is widely considered to be the father of aerobics and has written several books on the subject. His Bedrock Principle #1 states that almost everyone should engage in regular, moderate aerobic exercise. He says, 'The overwhelming weight of scientific evidence demonstrates conclusively that abandoning a sedentary lifestyle and following a moderate exercise routine will greatly reduce your risk of dying from all causes—and enhances your chance of living a longer, more active life.' (See Appendix VI for a detailed explanation of how oxygen is used for energy by the working muscles.)

In 1969, Jacki Sorensen pioneered aerobic dance in an air force base in Puerto Rico for army wives. Judie Sheppard Missett from Illinois combined her love for jazz and dance to put together Jazzercise, another form of aerobic dance exercise that includes some amount of weight training with dumb-bells and resistance bands. Jane Fonda, the film star, model, writer and activist, made aerobics hip and cool beginning in 1982. A huge female fan following popularized exercise, making it fashionable to be fit not just skinny. With her sexy leotards, leg warmers and high-energy dance routines Fonda took aerobics to a new level of enthusiasm and glamour.

The word 'aerobics' came about when the gym instructors got together and said: if we are going to charge $10 an hour, we can't possibly call it 'jumping up and down'.

—*Rita Rudner*

Gin Miller, creator of Step Reebok, started the trend of step classes. Steppers were introduced into every aerobic studio and various class formats including weights and barbells were incorporated. These aerobic classes were more athletic.

Billy Blanks developed tae-bo, a form of cardio kick-boxing based on Taekwondo, which went on to be a great commercial success. Kick-boxing is a fitness craze that is still very popular as a high-energy, calorie-burning workout.

Then came the Zumba craze in the mid 1990s. Beto Parez, a Latin American aerobic instructor, quite accidentally developed this Latin dance-based format of cardio. He apparently forgot his regular aerobic music at class one day and used his own music with his own choreography to go with the Latin beat. This was soon to grow into a worldwide craze.

In the early days not much was known about the ill effects of **high-impact** aerobics. Since most of the classes were designed with high-impact jumps and bounces, aerobics received a bad rap for being the cause of knee injury and so forth. It was believed that to be effective and high intensity, the workout needed to be high-impact. As research and awareness grew, however, workouts have been modified today to include more low-impact moves, which are not necessarily low in intensity. A step workout, for instance, can be made very high in intensity by increasing the height of the step, and by adding arm movements without adding impact or jumping.

Today, there are various forms of aerobic activities that you can opt from—new, emerging and interesting group classes like dancercise, hip-hop, belly dancing, pole dancing, and even desi versions of dance aerobics involving Bollywood and bhangra, which appeal to the Indian psyche. Each type of activity requires a different set of skills and a whole lot of coordination, reflexes, an ear for music and a sense of rhythm. This is not to say one can't learn on the job. All one requires is a good instructor willing to teach and correct.

WOMEN AND GROUP CLASSES

Women, particularly, benefit greatly from the social nature of a group class with its energy and camaraderie. They seem to enjoy it more than their male counterparts. Your chances of staying with an exercise programme are increased when you commit to a class with fixed timings, make social contacts, enjoy the sessions and see it more as fun rather than exercise. All this is, provided you can commit to a specific time every day.

Much of the popularity of the class has to do with the instructor and the bond she is able to create with her students. A knowledgeable, well-informed instructor will go a long way in helping the student grow in fitness. It is important that she is also able to anticipate and prevent injury or bad forms of exercise, and encourage the student to remain motivated with their fitness routine. She should be able to modify the same class for various levels of students. A low-impact version of the same move would spare the joints of an overweight or older individual. The focus has to be on the student and how she copes with the workout. It takes a highly skilled instructor to be able to inspire, correct and urge students to improve themselves without making them nervous or self-conscious.

Aerobic classes improve coordination and bring several muscle groups into play. Learning the steps motivates the students further. Such classes help enhance memory, reflexes and various motor neuron skills.

A group class can work in two ways:
- Either the student can be terribly motivated by both the instructor and other students, and constantly tries to improve herself,

- Or she could disappear in the group, blend into the background, and never really improve her intensity, technique or form.

EXERCISE CAUTION!

Words of caution, however, when new to a particular kind of activity: join a beginner's class where you will be taught modifications and choreography that is broken down. Learn the technique and build a strong foundation before attempting to move to more advanced classes. You could injure yourself if you are not well coordinated or balanced in your enthusiasm to keep up with the class or the instructor. Many of the classes presume you have the muscle strength and body awareness not to injure yourself by performing an awkward move.

From a trainer's perspective, while teaching a class one is constantly surprised at just how lacking in body awareness an individual can be, especially one who is not used to physical activity. So, for instance, in an aerobic class, a complicated choreography routine with jump squats, grapevines, step touches, lunges, jazz squares, shuffles and hip shakes would require you to know the basics of balancing your body and its centre of gravity to move smoothly from one step to another without looking plain silly and, more importantly, without injuring yourself. If a student has participated in sport, games and dance in her youth, chances are she still has **muscle memory**. Her body can be retrained more easily. However, someone who has been completely sedentary will find it that much harder to teach the body to move correctly.

Alternatively you can try walking, running, cycling, or cross-training if you so choose, either in a gym setting or outdoors. These are usually solo activities. Of course, you can always organize a walking or running group to keep motivation levels high. Such activities can be adjusted in one's routine with flexibility and allow to modify one's own intensity, duration and frequency of cardio. The disadvantage, of course, is the higher level of motivation required to just get on a treadmill and do your thing. The choice of activity depends on your own **fitness personality**.

I would recommend mixing activities while enjoying the available options to keep boredom at bay, and challenging your body differently.

> As you get fitter, it gets easier to include various forms of exercise and experiment with different classes.

PLAYING A GAME

One has to get fit for a game. Not everyone is a natural like Leander Paes, Nadia Comaneci or Michael Jordan. Even these famous and gifted stars train very hard to get fitter for their specific sport.

I know of several people who go out there and start playing a sport, unconditioned and unfit for it, and come back injured. **You have to get fit for the game, not expect the game to make you fit.**

In most fast-paced sports or games, one is required to be agile with the ability to move in several directions, stop abruptly, lean at different angles, execute lateral movements, jump, twist, bend, basically do everything the body is supposed to be able to do but cannot! It's a pity. We stop using our bodies and limit our physical movement to the extent that even something as simple as bending down to pick up a ball becomes a potential injury waiting to happen.

So if you decide to experiment with a game late in your life, I suggest you train for the various movements the game entails. I also suggest you train to strengthen your core, your back and the muscles around your knees to prevent untoward damage to these body parts.

**Watch Out for
Repetitive Stress Injury or RSI**

Performing the same movement repetitively can cause repetitive stress injury or RSI. The constant stepping in a step class, the continuous high-impact running motion while running, or performing an awkward movement with the hips, legs or shoulders while in an aerobic, hip-hop or Zumba class, can lead to **RSI**. Even sitting in front of the computer typing all day can cause RSI in the wrist, elbow or shoulder, not to mention neck strain, eye strain and a myriad other things.

In order to **prevent RSI**, the muscles should be strong and capable of the continuous imposition of movement. To avoid this type of injury, you need to strengthen the relevant muscles and work on your balance and flexibility simultaneously. So for example:

- A step class would require that you strengthen your thigh muscles to avoid impact and injury to the knee joint while stepping.
- You will need to train your core selectively while participating in a tae-bo class to be able to balance your body weight during the kicks and jumps.

Here is why it is important to incorporate all the 4 pillars of fitness. You might think you are doing just fine taking an aerobics class 6 days a week. Yes, you may be burning calories and staying slim. Ask yourself: are you strong and flexible as well? Is your diet providing you with the necessary nutrients now and for the future? Do you get enough rest so you are gaining the most out of your diet and exercise?

CARDIO FOR STAMINA

So, how do you go about planning your cardio? Do you jump in and take the most popular class in town because your best friend is doing it? Do you walk? Run? How do you plan your routine? How long should your cardio last on any given day? How hard should you work out?

The basic principles to follow while doing cardio are given below. Together they make up the **FITT principle**.

F—Frequency of cardio—how often

I—Intensity of cardio—how hard

T—Time—how long

T—Type of activity—what to do

How Often?

You should attempt to do your cardio at least 4 times a week for health purposes, more if the objective is weight loss.

According to the American surgeon general's statement: 'A mandatory minimum requirement just to maintain health fitness standards is regular, physical exercise for 30 minutes most days of the week, burning at least 150 calories per session or 1,000 calories per week and 2 sessions of strength training a week. Most people fail to meet even these basic health requirements.'

The Indian recommendation is 30 minutes a day, 5 days a week at a vigorous intensity.
Strength training of 1-3 sets of 8-12 repetitions (muscle mass building routine) 2-3 times per week.

Answer the Following Question:

How many times a week do **you** do cardio?
- 1-2 days/week
- 3-4 days/week
- 5-6 days/week

If you are overweight, you should have ticked 5-6 days per week. If you are of normal weight, you should have ticked 3-4 days per week. There is no place for 1-2 days per week!

People who participate in occasional exercise, often called the **weekend warriors**, are more prone to injury as a result of sudden bursts of intense activity.

It is better to do a little every day rather than a lot on one or two days.

How Hard?

The cardio intensity for weight loss can improve

heart 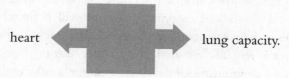 lung capacity.

For weight loss alone, a low intensity, routine workout is adequate, for all you need is to burn the adequate amount of calories. Remember that you will take much longer to burn the same number of calories working at a lower intensity. When you are overweight and unfit, it is much more difficult to increase your intensity. It is acceptable to stay at a lower intensity in the initial stages.

As you lose weight and improve in fitness, and if you want to improve the condition of your heart and lungs, you need to work at a higher intensity where you challenge the heart and lungs, get breathless, find it difficult to talk, and get your heart beating faster and stronger.

Monitoring your heart rate by counting your pulse rate is a scientific but somewhat difficult method of evaluating your intensity while working out. I find clients can barely count their pulse while seated or resting so the question of attempting it while working out is debatable. However, it is worthwhile learning how to count your pulse and keeping track of it.

Exercise that does not raise your heart rate to a certain level, and maintain it there for at least 20 minutes will not contribute significantly to cardiovascular fitness. So, for instance, I am often told by women that they do all the work in the house *that the maid doesn't do*, which is in essence cooking, perhaps folding clothes, setting dinner, feedings kids, walking around the house, watching TV, and so on. **This does not count for exercise, but is considered as activity.** Those women who do a lot more physical work around the house like vacuuming, laundry, swabbing floors and carrying groceries will definitely burn calories to help maintain weight. Since it is unlikely that your heart rate remains elevated consistently during housework, which is a prerequisite for developing cardiovascular endurance, such activity will do nothing for it.

Never underestimate the importance of daily activity in **weight management**, however. The secret of slim people is their ability to stay in constant motion! They are just more active through the day, doing little physical things, like rearranging their desk.

For something to be called **cardiovascular exercise**, on the other hand, it has to be consistent, structured and repetitive, using the major muscles of the body, maintaining an elevated heart rate at one's target heart rate or THR for a stipulated period of time.

How to increase intensity: I know you must wonder why one would want to increase the intensity of exercise in order to feel uncomfortable. The secret is, as one's fitness levels improve, one truly begins to enjoy the higher intensity workouts. The challenge, the sweat—*yes, even the sweat!*—and the breathlessness. Masochistic? The high after the workout is well worth the effort.

The intensity of any workout can be increased or decreased as required. While walking or running, increasing speed or incline will automatically increase intensity.

In a group fitness class, adding a larger range of movement, bigger arm circles, higher knee raises, or squatting lower, or adding a jump, thereby increasing impact as well, can increase the intensity of the very same workout. An experienced exerciser can modify her workout and manipulate intensity to her advantage as required. An experienced instructor can modify her class to suit various levels of students.

There are three ways of measuring the intensity of your workout to determine how hard you are working:

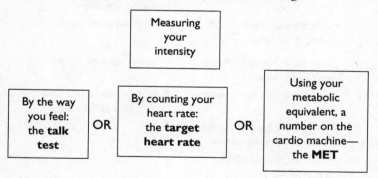

A simple subjective way to measure your intensity is the **talk test**. Gunnar Borg came up with a scale from 0–10 or 20 to measure how you feel during your workout. This gives you an idea of how hard you are working. The talk test assesses what is called your **rate of perceived exertion** or **RPE**, which is denoted on the **Borg scale**.

While working out you need to be able to talk but not sing! As you progress, you emerge into a zone where you can just about respond to conversation. Or construct a short sentence. At this point, you will be working at approximately 70 per cent of your intensity—or 7 on the 10-point scale.

0-10 Borg Rating of Rate of Perceived Exertion	Examples of Activity/Exercise
0	Resting, comfortable, inactive	Relaxing, watching TV
1	Relaxed and comfortable, can maintain this pace all day	Watching TV, chatting
2	Easy	Sitting at the desk working, talking
3	Moderate, feel could carry on, sweating a little	Doing small things around the house like dusting, folding clothes
4	Sort of hard, breathing harder	Heavier work like vacuuming, sweeping, cleaning
5 6	Fairly difficult, but can talk, slightly breathless	Moderate-paced walking.
7	Really hard, can still talk but don't really want to	Walking uphill or jogging
8	Really hard, can say a word or two only	Running much faster, walking briskly on a steep incline
9	Really, really hard—feel like you are probably going to die	Sprint
10	Maximum, all-out effort— already dead.	

Guess the intensity: In a group class, students are made to recite a few lines of a known rhyme or song to assess if they are working at their desired intensity. If they can sing it quite comfortably, or even sing along with the music in the background perhaps, obviously, they need to work harder. If they find it difficult to even squeak out a few words, then they need to cut back on intensity. An experienced exerciser knows innately just how hard to push herself without having to sing, talk or recite poetry. Until you reach that point, however, it is advisable to keep a track of your intensity.

The talk test, although still extensively used, often has inexperienced clients overestimating their intensity and ending up not pushing themselves to the best of their capability. Now we have a more objective way of assessing intensity in a gym setting called the MET, which is available on most gym equipment.

The heart rate you should maintain during your workout is called your **target heart rate (THR)**. There are several ways of arriving at this figure. One of the simplest is:

Maximum Heart Rate = 220 Minus Your Age

Your THR should be 50-80 per cent of your maximum heart rate depending on your fitness level.

If you are 30 years old, your maximum heart rate is 220 – 30 = 190.

Your 50 per cent intensity is 95 bpm. Your 70 per cent intensity is 133 bpm. As a beginner you therefore need to work between 50-60 per cent or 95-114 bpm.

An intermediate can work at 60-70 per cent or 114-140 bpm.

An advanced exerciser can work up to 80-90 per cent or 170 bpm.

A more complicated, but more accurate, method of evaluating intensity (see Appendix II) is using your **resting heart rate** (RHR). RHR should be determined by taking your pulse after sitting quietly for 5 minutes, or immediately on waking in the morning. An important application of your RHR is to assess fitness levels and overtraining. Keep a record of the RHR over a period of time.

- A falling RHR over time will indicate improved cardiovascular fitness levels.
- An increasing RHR over time will indicate overtraining or an illness.

Date ⇒	Today	Next Month	Following Month	And the Next Month
RHR ⇒				

When checking heart rate during a workout, take your pulse within 5 seconds after interrupting exercise because it starts to drop once you stop moving. Count the pulse for 10 seconds and multiply by 6 to get the per-minute rate.

MET or the **metabolic equivalent** is yet another very simple method of assessing your intensity. Most cardio machines in a gym setting, like the treadmill, elliptix and spin bike, will give you an indication of your working intensity through a number on the machine called the MET. For a given age and gender there is an optimum MET that one needs to try to achieve in order to improve cardiorespiratory endurance.

The energy expended at rest is generally referred to as 1 MET. As you increase physical activity your MET increases. Gardening, for instance, could have you working at a MET of about 4-5, depending on how hard you are digging. A stroll in the park could be anywhere from 3-5 MET. Showering, changing clothes, doing your hair getting from one room to another would be about MET 3. I suspect most of us stay at about a MET 1-3 all day long.

Extensive research done in the past evaluating the best workout intensities or METs for men indicated that if men worked out at their required MET, their chances of a **cardiovascular event—**like a **heart attack—was reduced by 75 per cent.** Similar contemporary research by Dr Martha Gulati and colleagues, done as late as 2005 on women, gives us similar information about the MET requirements for women.

The required MET is calculated depending on the age and basic lifestyle of the individual, whether sedentary or highly active. This is relevant only to physiologically normal people. Those with health issues, who are physically challenged or post surgery, are to be treated differently, and will have a different set of goals and working principles.

The formula commonly used to determine a woman's 100 per cent MET is:

$14.7 - (0.13 \times age)$

So, for instance, a 50-year-old woman's 100 per cent MET will be:

$14.7 - (0.13 \times 50) = 8.2$

8.2 will be the maximum MET she needs to attain. While working out she should aim to work from about 6 to 8.2 MET to maintain and improve the condition of her heart and lungs.

A fitness professional should be able to educate you on your required MET during your workout. Initially, achieving your required MET may seem a Herculean task. **You didn't quite anticipate how dreadful it would feel! How are you supposed to keep this up?** As your fitness levels increase, however, it gets easier and more manageable. It gives you a goal to work towards, which is easily measurable and reproducible since it is denoted by a simple number on your cardio machine. Most cardiovascular equipment in gyms have MET settings as an option on the control panel, and can be easily viewed while training.

You will notice that you can increase or decrease your MET by increasing the speed, incline or workload on the machine. Over a period, an experienced exerciser can easily recognize his working MET even while exercising outdoors without the aid of a machine.

You may not be able to sustain your required metabolic equivalent for the entire duration of your workout. The idea is to try to get to it from time to time. **In other words, push yourself beyond your comfort zone every few minutes during your workout to reach your required MET.**

The human body is enormously capable of improvement, provided we challenge it. Maintaining your intensity levels at a humdrum, comfortable level through your workout will only create monotony and set the stage for what is referred to as **hitting the wall** in physical fitness terms. You will see no progress.

On the other hand, being able to achieve your MET time and time again and being able to maintain it longer will give you a sense of achievement and satisfaction and will urge your body to higher limits.

If you happen to fall off the wagon and have not seen your training shoes in a while, it is always advisable to start over at a lower intensity and work your way up once again. Fitness levels tend to deteriorate with neglect. It is unrealistic and not very prudent to expect to resume where you left off after a long sojourn.

Of course there will be days when all you want to do is stroll, go through a gentle stretch class or practise relaxation. That's reasonable and acceptable. Let those days be few and far between.

Ways to increase your intensity, provided you can and there are no medical contraindications:

- Walk on an incline.
- Use bigger arm movements in an aerobic class.
- Use a higher step in a step class.
- Run instead of walk.
- Squat a little lower.
- Jump a little higher.

Short Bursts of Cardio Work Just as Well

When Megha joined TFL, she hated cardio. This was because she got so breathless that it was uncomfortable, and she would do anything to avoid the feeling. She would find any excuse to escape her cardio.

'Give me any amount of weight training,' she said, 'let me skip the cardio.' There was no doubt she was very good at weight training. Her form was excellent. She learnt the exercises quickly. Her strength improved in bounds.

She was well overweight, however, and needed to drop her fat percentage. Training with weights alone was insufficient. The calories she burnt at every workout session were insufficient to show any significant weight loss.

'Let's trick your body and mind into doing cardio,' I suggested. We came to a compromise.

We introduced short segments of cardio into her routine. She was instructed to walk as briskly as she could for 10 minutes 3 times a day. We then increased it to 10 minutes 4 times a day. Effectively, by the end of the second month, she was doing 40 minutes of cardio every day without even realizing it. She added walking on an incline. Something she was loath to do initially. She pushed her intensity to about 70 per cent. Since the segments of cardio were short, she was able to sustain the intensity and burn a fair number of calories collectively.

As her weight plummeted, she discovered the joy of cardio. It became easier and more enjoyable. She joined the step class, loved boot camp, continued to walk, and even tried Zumba, *though she...*

> ...*said she drew a line there!* Over 4 months she lost 14 kg and 6 per cent fat. Now she knows she has what it takes to have a complete routine including the weight training, cardio and stretches.

How Long?

Anywhere between 20 to 60 minutes depending on intensity and goals.

- Working at a higher intensity would mean you could keep your duration short and still burn the same number of calories.

- The duration need not be continuous. It has been found that even an accumulated sum of several bouts of exercise during the day is sufficient to reap the benefits of exercise. For those who find a long-drawn cardio routine of 40 minutes daunting, 2 sessions of 20 minutes will work just as well.

Abandon those excuses of lack of time. I am quite sure every one of us can manage 3 sessions of 15 minutes of cardio. We waste a lot of time in the course of the day that can be put to use effectively to get in a quick workout.

Those who have weight loss as a goal have to burn a large enough number of calories; therefore, a longer duration of cardio is required; 45-60 minutes 6 days a week is required initially.

For those individuals for whom the maintenance of fitness and weight is the objective, even a 20-30 minute cardio session 6 days a week should suffice. Increase your intensity, however, to 70-80 per cent, depending on whether you are a beginner or advanced exerciser.

WHAT KIND OF CARDIO ACTIVITY?

There are a variety of cardio activities to choose from. Everything depends on what you like to do and partly on your fitness personality. **My advice is to start with something simple like walking, then incline-walking, and then progress to running, dance aerobics, step classes, etc. Simultaneously strengthening the various muscles in the body will help you prevent injury during your cardio.**

Even if you choose to play a game like badminton as a form of cardio, it would be sensible to strengthen your legs and your core muscles for balance before, or at least simultaneously. Some of these games or classes call for the body to perform movements one is not accustomed to. For instance, how many of us step side to side (called lateral movement) on a daily basis? We most likely just walk or run, placing one foot in front of the other. This lateral movement, which is so commonly required in most games and aerobic classes, requires a great deal of balance and strength in the legs. It puts a tremendous amount of strain on the knee joint, which can result in injury to the knee unless the leg muscles are strong enough to take the impact. The sudden changes in direction, jumps to reach for the ball, stretches and twists require that you had better know your body well enough to know how to do what you are doing!

Walking	The simplest low-impact activity you can try. All of us learn how to walk, but do we walk right? Is it possible to walk wrong, you ask? Yes, it is. Your gait, or your method of walking is unique. Some have a very heavy footfall. Some are extremely light on their feet. Some appear to drag their weight from one foot to the other, not really lifting the body weight with the help of muscles.

Essentially, the strength of the leg muscles, calves, shins, thighs and buttocks, determines how you walk. Corrective exercises can help establish proper walking styles.

To increase intensity, walk on an incline. Incline-walking shapes and strengthens the large muscles of the lower body.

Living in Ooty has several advantages. We have natural inclines that are far more extreme than those found on any treadmill. It amuses me sometimes when, in my gym in Chennai, clients are shocked when I suggest a 15 per cent incline to improve their cardio.

'15 per cent? How can I walk on that kind of incline?' You can and people who live in hilly areas do, at probably 60 per cent inclines! It develops great, shapely legs. Now, want to give it a try?

Running	Running is a high-impact activity. The weight of the body pounding on the surface needs to be supported by the strength of the leg muscles. Else, the knee joint will take the strain. It is essential, therefore, for runners to strengthen the legs using weight-training exercises. Running can be a very high intensity exercise. **Wear specific running shoes for appropriate support.**
Elliptix	Sometimes called the cross-trainer, it uses the skiing motion. The machine needs to be made well to support body mechanics.
Rowing Machine	Another great piece of equipment to work your cardio. Involves the upper body and the core as well. Is low impact and fairly intense.
Stair Climber	Is a stepping machine. Great for the lower body. Often has a rowing action for the hands also.

Your other option, of course, is a group class. The key to group classes is the expertise and attitude of the instructor. A positive, exuberant instructor with a great sense of rhythm and energy can motivate even the most indolent students to get moving and sustain their fitness. It may be wise to choose your instructor carefully. Ask around, check for qualification and experience.

HOW TO OPTIMIZE YOUR CARDIO FOR FAT LOSS

*Please understand that before attempting techniques to increase fat loss by increasing intensity, you need to first and foremost **get your form of exercise right** at a lower intensity using basic moves, and then progress.*

In the gym	In a group class
Increase the intensity of your workout gradually till you are working at 70-80 per cent of your intensity. **Try varying the cardio machine.** In a gym setting, instead of using the treadmill all the time, try mixing it up with the spin bike, the elliptical trainer or the stepper. **Same activity, different intensity:** Even on the treadmill, don't go through the very same routine every single day. Your body tires of it easily; change your speed, increase the incline and/or duration with every workout. **Mix up your cardio with weights**: If you are scheduled to do a 30-minute cardio routine, start with 15 minutes of cardio at the highest intensity you can manage. Get off your cardio machine and complete your weight training for the day, then go back and complete the last 15 minutes of your cardio.	Attempt larger arm movements Squat lower Reach higher Lift the legs higher **You are in control of your intensity.** I see students in some classes repeat the same moves, mostly incorrectly, every session. You can increase the intensity to burn more calories and get the best from the class. If you have learnt a new step, go home and practise. It will add to the calories burnt during the day. **Try something new** to challenge your body when you are hovering on a plateau. There comes a time in everyone's fitness career when boredom sets in. You are absolutely tired of running or walking on the treadmill. Take a break from your usual activity and try something new for a change. You may choose not to pursue it, but at least it gives you the opportunity to experiment and prevents you from falling off the wagon.

Here are some of my favourite things—2 specialized workouts I love:

- High Intensity Interval Training or HIIT
- Boot Camp

These should not be tried unless you have been evaluated and have been prescribed the routines by a qualified professional and are properly guided. They are mostly for more advanced exercisers.

HIIT ON THE TREADMILL

This is an advanced technique used to burn the maximum number of calories for a minimum investment of time. It uses a combination of challenge and recovery cycles to burn calories and get a fantastic workout. The advantage of HIIT is that it trains the body to be capable of a higher level of intensity or, in other words, improves the **lactate threshold**. It can combine both cardio and weight training or cardio alone.

The high intensity aspect of the cycle causes the working muscles to work in the anaerobic zone. They are unable to use oxygen to function at that high level of intensity. As a result, they can continue to work at that intensity only for short bursts of time (about a minute). The muscles experience a burning when you are completely out of breath. You immediately move into the moderate intensity phase for the next 3-4 minutes, which is the time the muscles take to recover. This cycle can be repeated 3-4 times. Effectively, a HIIT routine does not take more than 20-30 minutes to complete. A HIIT routine essentially means that you intersperse very high intensity exercise—like sprinting in the anaerobic zone—with a lower level of activity (the aerobic zone).

A Sample Routine of an Advanced HIIT Training Schedule

Weeks ⇒	Warm Up and Dynamic Stretches	High Intensity Interval at Max Intensity Possible	Moderate Intensity Interval for Recovery 60-70 Per Cent	Number of Cycles	Cool Down and Static Stretches	Total Time Taken
First 2 weeks	5 minutes	20-30 second sprint	4.5-minute jog	X 3-4 cycles	5 minutes	25-30 minutes
Next 2 weeks	5 minutes	30-45 second sprint	3-minute run	X 3-4 cycles	5 minutes	Approximately 25 minutes
Next 2 weeks	5 minutes	45-60 second run at your maximum pace possible	4-minute jog at a much slower pace	X 4 cycles	5 minutes	30 minutes

ADVANTAGES OF HIIT

- A HIIT workout is **highly effective in burning fat**. It increases the number of calories you burn during the course of the workout and continues to burn a higher number of calories after the workout due to what is called an elevated EPOC—excess post-exercise oxygen consumption.

- **HIIT also leads to some metabolic adaptations** which make the body more efficient in utilizing fat as fuel. In other words, it helps burn fat more easily. HIIT can be attempted with any cardio equipment like the spin bike, stair climber, elliptix, and so on.

- **HIIT limits loss of muscle.** Due to the higher intensity and shorter duration of the workout, the loss of muscle is limited. Long-duration, steady-state cardio sessions such as long runs or walks tend to lead to muscle loss along with fat loss. Muscle loss, as we all know, has to be avoided at any cost especially as we age.

- **HIIT is extremely time effective:** When you have only 30 minutes at hand, a good HIIT can burn about 300-500 calories and continue to keep your metabolism elevated following your workout.

- **Prevents boredom:** Sometimes long-drawn cardio routines with repetitive motion can lead to boredom. There is absolutely no chance of encountering boredom with a HIIT where all you can think of is getting to the next stage!

PREREQUISITES FOR HIIT

HIIT should be done only about 2-3 times a week. Done every day, it can lead to overtraining and injury. It needs to be interspersed with lower intensity, longer-duration cardio routines. Being an advanced exercise format, HIIT requires training and proper guidance. It also requires a medical evaluation to rule out pre-existing cardiac problems, if you are capable of working out at 70-90 per cent of your maximum heart rate for about 20 minutes. If over the age of 40, a stress test would be mandatory.

TABATA

This is another interesting form of HIIT. Founded by a Japanese scientist called Izumi Tabata, it uses weights and cardio. It also has a very specific time format of 20 seconds of intense training + 10 seconds rest x 8 sessions = a total of 4 minutes.

A Tabata routine could look something like this:

Each column represents 20 seconds of the exercise + 10 seconds of rest.

Jumping jacks	Squats	Push-ups	Knee highs	Jumping jacks	Squats	Push-ups	Lunges

In 4 minutes, therefore, one can get a very high intensity workout. The cycle is usually repeated with different exercises for a total of about 12-15 minutes.

I don't think everyone can attempt these forms of exercise. I know they sound exciting and appealing, especially when they promise great results in such short periods of time. The point is, in order to get in a good HIIT you have to be of a certain level of fitness. You have to train at moderate intensities, strengthen your muscles with weight training, and then gradually introduce HIIT routines to challenge yourself. This way you not only enjoy the workout more, but also prevent injury and get the maximum benefits from the workout.

BOOT CAMP

Boot camp workouts are another interesting way of adding variety and challenging the body. As the name suggests, the exercise format originated in the US army. In essence, it consists of military style exercises, usually done outdoors, interspersed with some cardio work like short sprints, side shuffles or lunge walking. Some boot camp workouts can be very rough and strenuous. They can be modified, however, to suit individual needs and can even be conducted indoors to music.

Some of the main advantages of boot camp are that it involves simple exercises that almost anyone can do provided they are trained to do them. You don't require complicated equipment and you don't necessarily even need music.

Boot camp will certainly not appeal to everyone. It is hard-core fitness and can be very challenging. My students groan

---

An example of a boot camp routine could look like this:

1.	Warm up and dynamic stretch x 5-7 minutes
2.	Running x 3 minutes
3.	Push-ups x 20
4.	Squats x 20
5.	Jumping jacks x 40
6.	Running x 3 minutes
7.	Spiderman x 20
8.	Lunge walking x 20
9.	Push-ups x 20
10.	Running x 3 minutes
11.	Knee highs x 1 minute
12.	Jump squats x 20
13.	Spiderman x 20
14.	Jumping jacks x 40
15.	Side shuffles x 3 sets
16.	Running x 3 minutes
17.	Cool down and stretch x 5-7 minutes

when I start a boot camp routine, but by the end of it they are so thrilled to have completed it that it seems worth it, and they actually look forward to the next one!

Quick Facts about Cardio

- Cardiovascular exercise is any form of exercise that elevates the heart rate and gets you breathing hard to improve your stamina.

- This form of exercise strengthens the circulatory (heart and blood vessels) and respiratory (lungs) systems.

- Everyone requires cardio, even the slim ones. Only the duration, intensity and frequency will vary for each individual.

- **Intensity** can be measured by the **talk test**. A beginner can start at 4-6 on the Borg scale. Advanced exercisers work at 7 and progress at intervals to 8-9.

- **Duration and frequency:** Work towards getting in at least 20-30 minutes of cardio at least 4 days a week if you want to maintain fitness. An overweight individual can increase her workout to 45-60 minutes a day, 6 days a week, to lose fat.

- Keep a watchful eye on your **MET** which is yet another measure of intensity, evaluated easily on a cardio machine.

- If you persist at the same intensity, your fitness will not evolve. With time and improved fitness levels, you need to be able to increase your intensity comfortably. This is an indication of the improving condition of your heart and lungs.

- If you are unable to work out continuously for a longer period, **split sessions** of about 15 minutes, 3 times a day can also produce the necessary benefits.

- Incorporate various forms of cardio if you can, like flat walking, incline-walking, interval training, step class and dance aerobics, to add variety and keep boredom at bay.

- Advanced exercisers can include various forms of combination exercises that work different muscles, like HIIT (with challenge and recovery cycles) and boot camp.

Quick Look Table

TO DETERMINE WHAT YOU NEED TO DO DEPENDING ON YOUR GOALS

FITT Principle	For Weight Loss	To Maintain Health	To Improve Stamina
Frequency	6 days a week	4 days a week	4-5 days a week
Intensity	50-60 per cent	60-70 per cent	70-80-90 per cent
Time	60 minutes	45 minutes	30 minutes
Type	Any aerobic activity like walking, dance aerobics or cycling.	Any aerobic activity like walking, running, dance aerobics or cycling.	Change your activity so you do different things each time to add variety and to challenge yourself.

Questions & DIY

- Record your resting pulse at regular intervals.

- Which cardio options do you enjoy the most?
  ‣ Walking or running
  ‣ Aerobic dance
  ‣ Stepper
  ‣ Jazzercise or Zumba
  ‣ Cycling
  ‣ Others

- For how long do you do cardio every day?

- How many times a week do you do your cardio?

- How hard do you work out?
  ‣ I am very comfortable throughout my workout, I chat, sometimes hum along with the music, I hardly break a sweat.

> ▸ I am comfortable during most of my workout, but intermittently, I push myself to a point where I get breathless, can barely say a few words. I am sweating by the end of the workout.
>
> ▸ I am completely breathless throughout the workout. I am quite uncomfortable, sweat profusely and feel like my heart is going like a trip hammer. I literally punish myself!

- Plan 3 ways in which you can increase the intensity of your cardio.

- Plan your own boot camp routine to burn more calories.

- **Assess your stamina yourself.** Here's a table to give you an idea of where you stand. How long does it take you to walk a mile (1.6 km)? Can you take your pulse at the end of it?

Age ⇒	20-29	30-39	40-49	50-59	60-69	70+
Excellent	<13.12	<13.42	<14.12	<14.42	<15.06	<18.18
Good	13.12-14.06	13.42-14.36	14.12-15.06	14.42-15.36	15.06-16.18	18.18-20.00
Average	14.07-15.06	14.37-15.36	15.07-16.06	15.37-17	16.19-17.30	20.01-21.48
Fair	15.07-16.30	15.37-17	16.07-17.30	17.01-18.06	17.31-19.12	21.49-24.06
Poor	>16.30	>17.00	>17.30	>18.06	>19.12	>24

CHAPTER 6

PILLAR 2

MUSCLE STRENGTH

The human body is a consummate example of fine architecture. It is sacrilege to allow it to disintegrate into a poorly functioning disarray of accumulated fat, poor muscle mass, muscle imbalance, improper gait and ungainly posture. This only results in aches and pains and puts one's health at risk, depreciates your appearance and lowers self-esteem. Several issues, like muscle imbalance, poor posture, weak joints and poor strength, can be corrected with weight training in combination with a good cardio and flexibility routine.

How many of you have entered the weight room of a gym and felt like you have walked into a Japanese torture chamber with strange gadgets and gizmos? How many of you have felt an excruciating sense of inadequacy as you watched some gym rat squeeze under the hack squat machine, or another execute some impressive preacher curls? It's really not that complicated. The exercises are simple enough to learn and can even be enjoyable! The changing shape of your body is sufficient testimony and encouragement to keep you on the wagon even if the scientific corroboration for the benefits of weight training does not impress you.

> Our research shows that a program of strength training not only improves bone density, but reduces falls, improves arthritis symptoms, and increases flexibility and strength.
> — *Dr Miriam Nelson, director of the John Hancock Research Center and professor at the Friedman School in Tufts University*

WHAT REALLY HAPPENS WHEN YOU TRAIN WITH WEIGHTS?

Our entire body is encased with muscles. Muscles envelop our limbs, support our joints and protect out internal organs. **Muscles are the essence of movement.** The human body has about 640 muscles. Beautiful tiny ones like those around the eyes, which perform the intricate job of moving the eyeballs as you scan a menu or squint in the sun; large, powerful muscles like those of the back and legs, which power running, bending and twisting. When we talk about weight training, we are essentially training or building the major muscles of our torso, the back, chest, neck, abdomen, shoulders and our limbs—the arms and legs.

Each muscle or group of muscles enables a certain movement in the body. For instance, the bicep muscle in front of the upper arm causes the elbow to flex and the arm to bend. The gluteus maximus or the butt muscles facilitate the extension of the hip joint and the entire leg to move backward during the walking or running motion. Since the activation of a muscle or group of muscles leads to a certain movement, repeating that very movement using an external resistance, like dumb-bells, barbells or one's own body weight, will increase its size and strength, and improve its shape.

DOMS or Delayed Onset Muscle Soreness

When one trains a muscle with an external resistance, overcoming this external weight leads to small tears in muscle fibres. These tears heal to form stronger bonds. This healing process, which occurs over 24 to 48 hours following the training session, causes a dull aching sensation in the worked muscle called DOMS or delayed onset muscle soreness.

I know women who stop training when they experience DOMS because they believe it is an indication that something is terribly wrong. Nothing is wrong, your muscles are responding, growing and getting stronger. Persist with your workout and you will achieve the body you always dreamt of.

Taking a warm bath has been found to ease DOMS. According to some studies, stretching does not appear to minimize the symptoms, but conventionally, stretches and warm showers are advised.

Continue to exercise as per schedule. Missing your regular routine will only delay recovery and prevent you from acclimatizing to the stress on the muscles.

Lactate Threshold

Weight training is an anaerobic form of exercise. The intensity of the exercise is high. The muscles, therefore, use the anaerobic metabolic pathway to generate energy. This pathway is independent of the supply of oxygen because oxygen cannot be supplied fast enough for such intensity of action. As a result, the metabolic by-product of this pathway is an accumulation of lactic acid within the muscles. Have you experienced the excruciating burning sensation in the muscles towards the end of a set of repetitions of an exercise? A point at which you just cannot lift that dumb-bell one more time! This is your lactate threshold. This threshold is determined by how competent your muscle is in the anaerobic metabolic pathway and how rapidly your body is able to remove the waste product of lactic acid. If you are unable to do this effectively, you will experience a great deal of discomfort shortly into higher intensity exercise, and be forced to stop. If your body is efficient at generating energy and force without the supply of oxygen and at removing these waste products, then you will be able to exercise for a much longer period.

The lactate threshold can be reached rapidly even with very high intensity cardio. Sprinting, for instance, uses the anaerobic metabolic pathway, and 30-90 seconds into the sprint you will find you are unable to sustain that level of speed and intensity.

To increase your lactate threshold, you have to train at higher levels of intensity at least a few days in the week.

MUSCLE IMBALANCE

One can address specific body parts that are weak, have poor muscle mass or are imbalanced by training specific muscles. Most muscles exist in pairs, one on either side of the body. Sometimes, the muscles on one side of the body may be stronger, weaker or less flexible than their corresponding pairs, creating an imbalance. This could lead to various problems including poor posture, improper gait or even pain. Poor hamstring strength, for instance, is a common cause of back pain and injury. Weight training can be designed in such a way that such problems may be avoided and treated.

COMMON MISCONCEPTIONS SURROUNDING WOMEN AND WEIGHTS

I will look masculine: The truth is, it is not easy to **bulk up**. It takes hours of advanced exercise routines to get to the bodybuilder status. Recreational weight training cannot achieve such immense proportions. The male hormone testosterone aids in the increase in muscle size. There are specific training protocols to achieve size and others to achieve **tone or strength**. Depending on exactly what you are hoping to achieve, you can have a routine designed specifically for you.

Mira is 55 years old. She is slightly built on a slim frame and most women her age and size would have been happy to remain that way. However, Mira was sure she did not want to be slim and have poor muscle, especially as she aged.

'If I allow myself to gain fat and lose muscle with age like most women do, that's where I will be,' she said.

She trains very seriously with weights every day. Her routine may put many men to shame. She often hears a male gym rat wondering, 'What is she trying to prove?'

'I am not trying to prove anything,' says Mira. 'I just want my body to remain firm, toned and completely functional for as long as possible.' She is gorgeous at 55. Her body can pass for 20 years younger. She is far from masculine. In her silk saris, she is the epitome of a gracious Indian woman, but one of steel.

Weight training is what keeps her that way. Her cardio is only for maintenance—20 minutes 3 to 4 times a week at a high intensity. Her flexibility was lacking, however. I put her on to a stretching routine a few times a week. Her flexibility and balance have now improved and she is thrilled to have something new to work on.

If I stop training, the muscle will turn into fat: Muscle and fat are two entirely different types of tissue, like chalk and cheese. One cannot turn into the other. When women or men stop a weight-training programme, they start to lose muscle mass due to inactivity and disuse. They most often also stop watching their diet. The combination of poor eating habits and the fact that their metabolism and calorie expenditure have diminished due to inactivity causes an accumulation of fat, giving the impression that the subject's muscle is being turned into fat, while in reality muscle is lost and fat accumulates.

As long as I am training, I can eat whatever I want: The nutritional equation works on the principle that calories consumed need to equate approximately the calories expended in order to maintain your weight. If calories consumed exceed the calories burnt, the result is weight gain in the form of fat accumulation. This implies that when you train with weights and are burning excess calories, you can afford to increase calorie intake. Unless you want to lose excess fat, in which case you need to go into a calorie deficit.

You cannot eat whatever you want, however. Training does not grant you license for greed. The interesting thing is that when you train, you tend to eat healthy. You are more discerning and often in a better frame of mind.

If I train with weights, I don't need to do cardio: Stamina, Strength, Endurance and Flexibility are the 4 crucial pillars of a sound fitness programme. The combination and ratio of weight training to cardio and flexibility may change depending on the goals and objectives of the individual. An underweight person, for instance, requires a heavier and longer weight-training routine with a shorter cardio session. A person wanting to lose fat would need to use lighter weights, more repetitions with very little rest between sets, and a longer cardio session.

Cardio trains the heart, lungs and blood vessels—the

cardiovascular system; while weight training addresses the muscles, tendons and ligaments—the musculoskeletal system. Both aspects are equally important.

Weight training will make me stiff and muscle-bound: Not if you include adequate flexibility in your routine, which is a significant component of a good fitness routine. The flexibility of individual muscles is enhanced by deliberately stretching the muscle in a controlled manner after every exercise session. Modalities like yoga will further improve flexibility. This misconception arises because it is believed that a bodybuilder who trains with weights must be inflexible, and therefore weight training will make you inflexible. Neither is true. Bodybuilders who are sound in their knowledge of bodybuilding technique and principles will always include some serious stretching in their routine. The flexibility of world-class bodybuilders is proof of what the body is capable of.

I should not weight-train because I have cervical spondylosis, back pain, knee pain: This is a very common misconception. There are certain movements that one should refrain from in the above conditions, but, by and large, the importance of weight training remains even for those with the above problems as for those without, in fact more so. You can work around the problem.

Knee and back pain are very often the result of poor and weak muscles surrounding those joints. By strengthening those very muscles, you can support weak knees or an unstable back. One can always circumvent the current problem and strengthen muscles and body parts surrounding and supporting the weakened part. The concerned body part can then be addressed once one is ready, both physically and psychologically.

I cannot weight-train if I have high blood pressure as it will further elevate my blood pressure: When weight training is taught correctly and executed faultlessly, your blood pressure will not be affected. The problem arises when women are confused about the technique of breathing and lifting. Many tend to hold their breath in an effort to lift the weight. This manoeuvre, called the Valsalva manoeuvre, could potentially increase blood pressure.

This is one of the reasons I believe weight training has to be taught very precisely. There are so many things you could do wrong and end up hurting yourself. Do understand, it is not the exercise that is to be blamed, but the way it is performed.

BENEFITS OF WEIGHT TRAINING

- Developing better **shape and structure:** Indulging in cardio alone may aid weight loss resulting in decreased size, but the shape of the body barely changes. Individual parts of the body can be addressed with weight training to either lean the muscle or increase the muscles mass as required.

- **Firms and tones** the body and prevents ungainly sagging of bodily parts, giving it a more youthful appearance.

- The right training protocol will improve **muscular strength.** Which woman wouldn't like to be stronger?

- **Improves balance** by increasing the strength of appropriate muscles in the legs and core. The consequence of this improved balance is a decreased incidence of falls and injury, particularly in the elderly.

- **Essential for women:** Prevents and treats a predominantly women's disease, **osteoporosis**, by increasing the mineral deposits of the bones and strengthening the joints.

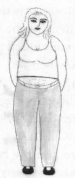
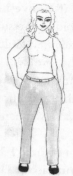
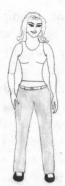

| Excess Fat | Only Cardio | Cardio + Weight Training + Balanced Diet |

- Improves **self-esteem, confidence and mood**. Of course, you are more confident with your sleek and firm body!

> **Weight Training Aids Fat Loss:** The average woman who strength-trains 2 to 3 times a week for 2 months will gain nearly 1 kg muscle and will lose 1.5 kg fat. As your lean muscle increases, so does your resting metabolism and you burn more calories all day long. Generally speaking, for each half kilo of muscle you gain, you burn 35 to 50 more calories each day. This adds up to a formidable number of burnt calories in the long run.

- **Protects against back injury, pain and arthritis:** Strength training not only builds stronger muscles but stronger connective tissue surrounding the muscles, tendons and ligaments, which then protect vulnerable parts of your body like the back and knees.
- **A younger, firmer body:** Weight training is a great way to **delay the ageing process**, even reverse it if started as late as in the seventies.
- **Important for diabetics:** Weight training **improves insulin sensitivity** and **fat oxidation**, thereby helping

in the better control of diabetes. Regular weight training has been found to **keep blood sugar** on an even keel. Diabetics who train with weights have better prospects at managing their disease, even reducing their dosage of medication.

- You will also **reduce your risk of heart disease** by lowering bad cholesterol and raising good cholesterol. These benefits may be maximized by including cardio along with your weight training.

GOAL SETTING

Most often, a professional and an exercise strategist can aid goal setting. Most women don't know what they need or what goals to set. We, at TFL, usually sit with a client to discuss her problems, and then work towards the solutions and goals.

Before you start training with weights, set a goal or several goals. Decide what you want to get out of your workout. Are you lifting weights to improve daily functionality? Health? Appearance? Or sports performance? Once this has been determined, your routine can be better tailored specifically for you by choosing exercises that will target the proper muscles. Specific goals could include improving knee strength or rehabilitating the back to manage back pain. You could train to improve posture by correcting muscle imbalance.

> When Kiran first came to see me, she was a slim waif of a girl with a pixie face and cheeky grin. She was keen on 'gaining weight the healthy way'. Her father had read my article in the newspaper that discussed the importance of weight training for women, and had decided that his daughter needed it. I was impressed. Not many men of that generation were convinced about weight training, let alone for their daughters.

Kiran started training with us at the fitness studio. Her first couple of months consisted of getting accustomed to handling the weights and understanding how to eat better. She is a vegetarian like many Indians. Her diet consisted primarily of carbs from the bread/cereal group. If it wasn't yogurt and rice, it was potatoes, pongal or idlis. She essentially consumed as many as 10-12 servings of the bread/cereal group in a day. There was barely any protein, however. The lentils she ate were minimal. She disliked soy or soy products; she didn't eat eggs; occasionally, she munched on nuts. Of course, there were the usual indulgences with sinful Indian sweetmeats, biscuits, cookies, cakes, chocolates, etc. It was a disaster. She was underweight but definitely not healthy.

Over the months, she learnt to understand food groups and tried to include as many vegetarian protein options in her diet as possible. She started drinking soymilk, increased her intake of lentils. She cut down on her bread/cereal group, snacked on nuts and sprouts, and ate more fruit.

Most impressive of all, she trained seriously with weights. She could bench-press 18 kg and bicep curl 7. She loved the yoga routines we did. Her back bend was impressive.

Today she is proud of her body. She is also certain she will not tread the same path as her mother who had been a waif like the daughter in her youth, but who has grown to ample proportions and is now heading towards a knee replacement.

BASIC PRINCIPLES OF WEIGHT TRAINING

Nothing looks worse than poor training technique!

One of the most valuable lessons to learn in the initial stages of your weight-training career is proper form and technique. Weight training is based on the scientific principles of human anatomy and physiology. If you have no experience with weights, invest a couple of months with a personal trainer until you are familiar with the drill, and terms like 12 rep max, super-setting, keep the knees soft, circuit training, etc. don't sound like an alien language. It is absolutely crucial to adhere to proper form and technique to prevent injury. After all, you are handling external weights. Most women are accustomed to not more than a broom or a laptop, both of which come feather-light these days. In the initial stages, I see some struggling even with 1-kg dumb-bells for their shoulder press, or grimacing through a mere couple of push-ups with incredulous looks of pure agony on their faces! Then, of course, they build in strength and grow in confidence. It is thrilling to watch them get excited with their own achievements and growth.

The proper alignment of the spine and joints, immaculate execution of movement and proper breathing technique are vital in preventing injury. Weight training should be taught by a patient and experienced instructor. It would save you a lot of trouble if you spent time learning every single exercise you are supposed to do to absolute precision, initially. Be obsessed if you must.

Breathing is probably one of the most important aspects of weight training.

Remember!
Breath Out (Exhale) on Exertion.

For example, if you are executing a bicep curl, you breathe out as you flex your elbow and lift the weight towards your shoulder—the **concentric phase of the exercise**—and breathe in as you lower the weight, called the **eccentric phase of the exercise**.

The worst thing you can do is to hold your breath while training. Get your breathing right first before you progress to higher weights or more advanced exercises.

Never work the same muscle group within 48 hours.

Work opposing muscles—biceps and triceps, pecs (chest) and lats (back). It is not mandatory that they need to be worked in the same session. Just remember to fit them in and balance your workout during the course of the week.

Always stretch after a session to keep the muscles supple and prevent pain and injury.

Rest and nutrition *cannot be overemphasized*. The building of the muscle occurs not during the actual course of the workout, but during the rest period. Ensure at least 8 hours of sleep to gain the maximum benefits of weight training. Following a healthy balanced diet is important to keep the muscles nourished.

Move slowly: It is pointless to cheat yourself by racing mindlessly through your exercises. Take about 3 seconds to contract the muscle, hold the contraction for another second or two, and then release to a count of 4 seconds. This time-breakdown will maximize strength gain. Remember to exhale as you contract the muscle.

Overload principle: Feel the burn! In order to build muscle strength and size you need to challenge it more than it is accustomed to. In other words, when you train, you need to overload your muscle and the last few repetitions of each set should be completed only with difficulty. The weight you use has to be heavy enough for it to work in building that muscle. If the weight is too light and you are swinging it around easily or could even complete a few more reps than the set calls for, then the weight is obviously insufficient. You need to **feel the burn** while performing the last 2-3 reps.

The burning sensation in the working muscle is due to the accumulation of lactic acid in it. A few seconds of rest will wash away this metabolic by-product and you will (surprisingly) be able to do your next set when you think you should be retiring for the day.

Progression of weight: To avoid muscle adaptation or stagnation you need to keep challenging it every few weeks by changing the intensity. You could change the number of reps, sets or the weight used depending on your goals. If you continue to participate in the same workout week after week, you **hit a plateau.** Nothing changes. You see no improvement.

Sequence of exercises: The body is divided into various body parts. The entire chest, for example, is considered one unit although it comprises of more than just one muscle, which is popularly known as the 'pecs'. So, usually, one body part is exercised on any one given day. Depending on the time available for weight training, one can incorporate as many body parts as possible into one day's routine.

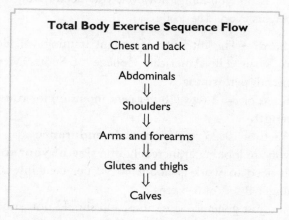

Total Body Exercise Sequence Flow

Chest and back
⇓
Abdominals
⇓
Shoulders
⇓
Arms and forearms
⇓
Glutes and thighs
⇓
Calves

While training, one must follow a sequence of exercises. Start with the larger muscles and follow up with the smaller ones. In other words, start with the central muscles in the body and move towards the periphery. For instance, if one is working

the chest, back, shoulders and arms on any given day, start with
the chest or back. Follow up with the shoulders and complete
the routine with the arms and then the forearms. The basic
premise behind this principle is that if the arms (the smaller
muscles) are used and exhausted first, then performing the
exercises for the shoulders (the larger muscles) is compromised,
since the arms which are brought into play while training the
shoulders have already been fatigued.

Consistency is the key. Once you commit to weight training,
persist with it. Resist the urge to skip sessions. **If you can't
do a lot, do a little,** for a shorter session is better than none
at all.

How often?—It is sufficient to weight-train 2-3 times a week.
Address all the muscle groups to balance your routine. If your
objective is bodybuilding, however, you need to be training
with weights every day.

How hard?—The intensity of weight training will depend
on your goals. The American College of Sports Medicine
recommends performing
* 4-6 sets of 8-12 reps (70 per cent intensity) for **muscular
  strength**
* 1-3 sets of 10-25 reps for **muscle endurance**
* If you are looking at increasing the **size of your muscle**,
  you need to work at about 80-90 per cent intensity by
  doing 4-8 sets of 6-8 reps.
These are just general suggestions, and should not to be used
unless prescribed by a qualified professional.

How do you evaluate the intensity of weight training?
Intensity is the number of repetitions of the exercise that you
can complete with good form with a given weight. So, for

instance, if you are able to complete 12 bicep curls using 4-kg dumb-bells, your intensity is about 70 per cent. It has been found that '12 rep max', or the amount of weight you lift in order to perform 12 repetitions, is your 70 per cent intensity. If you increase the weight to 5 kg, however, you may be able to complete only 10 repetitions with good form. You are then working at approximately 80 per cent intensity. Scale up the weight used and you will be able to perform fewer repetitions.

How long?—If you are participating in only 2 sessions per week and addressing all the body parts on both days, your routine will probably last about 40 minutes. You could, however, do 4 20-minute sessions per week instead. A very basic and quick weight-training routine can be completed in 20 minutes. The following suggestions depend on the number of days you are willing to train. The number of sets, reps and the weight used, of course, will have to be determined separately.

6 Days a Week Routine

Monday: Chest and Back + Upper and Lower Abs

Tuesday: Glutes, Legs and Obliques

Wednesday: Shoulders and Arms + Upper and Lower Abs

Thursday: Chest and Back + Obliques

Friday: Glutes and Legs + Upper and Lower Abs

Saturday: Shoulders and Arms + Obliques

4 Days a Week Routine

Monday: Chest, Back, Shoulders and Arms

Tuesday: Glutes, Legs and Abs

Thursday: Chest, Back, Shoulders and Arms

Friday: Glutes, Legs and Abs

---

3 Days a Week Routine

Monday: Chest, Back and Arms

Wednesday: Whole Body

Friday: Legs, Glutes and Abs

2 Days a Week Routine

Monday: Whole Body

Thursday: Whole Body

SPECIFIC ISSUES FOR WOMEN TRAINING WITH WEIGHTS

- The **Q angle** is the angle between the straight line from the patella or kneecap to the ground, and the direction of the quadriceps muscle. This is larger for women, and is due to their wider hips. It could put a strain on the knee joint, for women doing the narrow squat.

- The **vastus medialis** or **the inner part of the quadriceps** muscle is sometimes weaker in women and needs to be specifically trained.

- Women may have **lax joints** especially after childbearing.

- Their **pelvis may be tilted inordinately** forward following pregnancy, and needs to be watched and corrected.

- The **lumbar area of the spine may be arched** inward for many women, especially if they are constantly on high heels. This can cause lower back and calf muscles to be excessively tight.

- **Low back exercises** are as important as abdominal exercises to balance the muscles.

- Women usually have **poorer upper body strength** due to less muscle mass and lack of strengthening or use of the muscles.

- Women tend to have more **postural problems** that need to be addressed with a proper strengthening schedule.

Because of the need for extra strength training as I grow older, I'm currently planning to add an extra day of weight work to my regimen.

—*Dr Kenneth Cooper, Father of Aerobics*

Pooja was an aerobic instructor. She taught 5-6 classes a week and made it a point to run 3 times a week on her own to keep her stamina levels elevated. I was concerned that she was not training with weights to strengthen her muscles. Her classes involved a lot of high-impact moves like jumps and, in addition, her own workout (the running) was yet another high-impact activity.

After 6 months of this, she began to feel pain in the left knee. She pushed through her pain, sometimes using a knee guard, reluctant to give up teaching. When I saw her she was in a lot of pain and her knee was swollen. A visit to an orthopaedist indicated that she may have a ligament injury and would need to rest.

She was eager to heal quickly. Her students missed her, she said. She needed to get back to working out ASAP.

'You can't speed up healing, Pooja,' I cautioned. We started with simple quad-squeezing exercises. She did them every day whenever she could. After a week of this, she started with light weights and included:
- Leg extensions to strengthen her quadriceps,
- Leg curls to strengthen her hamstrings,
- Calf raises to strengthen her calves,
- Foot extensions with the resistance band to strengthen her shin.

We also had her stretch for about 15 minutes every day.

She then started working on her upper body. She was surprised at how much she enjoyed weight training. The high was very different from the one you get after an intense cardio workout. That she was used to. It took some time for her to learn to slow...

...down, focus on the muscle she was working, and keep the fine balance between pushing too hard and doing too little.

This was 3 years ago. Today she trains regularly with weights to maintain strength. Her knee has healed and she is back to teaching aerobic classes 5 days a week. She loves her class, but knows that to maintain the balance she has to strength-train as well.

Own-body weight exercises: Strength, tone and muscle mass can also be achieved with own-body weight exercises, like the squat, push-up and tricep dip. The caveat for this kind of exercise is that you need to be capable enough of withstanding your own body weight. Unlike using an external weight like a dumb-bell, where the amount of weight used can be adjusted, one cannot alter one's body weight! In the initial stages of fitness, very often, one is not strong enough to accommodate one's own body weight.

The point is, your muscles should be strong enough to withstand your body weight. So either you need to lower your body weight or increase the strength of the muscles. Preferable to do both!

Own-body weight exercises are important for many reasons. They remind you to maintain a ceiling to your own weight. When you are unable to lift your own weight, you know you need to lose it and strengthen your muscles. These exercises allow for balance and core strength as well. Performing a push-up is not the same as a chest press. While both exercises essentially work the chest, triceps and front of the shoulders, with the chest press, you are lying on a bench, your back and core well supported, and performing the exercise; whereas with the push-up, you are lifting your own body weight with your chest, shoulders and triceps keeping the core engaged (tummy tucked in, back flat). Many more muscles are being engaged. Lastly, these exercises also work the cardiovascular system. Doing push-ups and squats gets you breathless, inciting the heart and lungs to work harder.

But you do **need some preparation before engaging in these exercises.** Strengthen each muscle individually. Do leg presses, leg extensions, leg curls first, training the hip, butt and the thighs for a couple of weeks, and then attempt the squats. This way your knees are spared the strain of the exercise because the leg muscles will do all the work. You can then move on to doing squats with weights, single leg squats, jump squats, and so on.

Here are some of my favourite things! Most often, I don't have time for long-drawn workouts. I always try to fit in as much as I can in the shortest time possible:

- Super-setting
- Circuit training
- Combination exercises

They should not be tried unless you have been evaluated and have been prescribed the routines by a professional and are properly guided. They are mostly for more advanced exercisers.

In order to train with weights and burn as much fat during the process as possible, the entire workout should be done without a break. Normally, sets are separated by a rest period of about 30-60 seconds depending on the weight used, during which the accumulated lactic acid is removed. In order to do a time-saving workout, the following methods are used.

Super-setting is a method by which two exercises are performed back-to-back without a rest period. These two exercises will address two antagonistic muscles. While one muscle is resting, you can work the antagonistic muscle, thereby saving time. The following exercises for the arms can be super-set, for example, bicep curls, followed by overhead tricep extensions, followed immediately by the next set of bicep curls. Continue in this vein till you complete the entire number of sets required. Move on to the next super-set which could be bicep hammer curl followed by tricep push down.

Circuit training is a method by which a whole series of exercises addressing various body parts is completed without a rest, then followed by the next round. The required number of sets are completed in circuits thereby wasting no time. For example, the following exercises for the **upper body** may be completed in a circuit:

Body Part	Circuit 1	Circuit 2	Circuit 3
Chest	Push-up 20	Push-up 20	Push-up 20
Back	Lat pulldown 15	Lat pulldown 15	Lat pulldown 15
Shoulder	Military press 15	Military press 15	Military press 15
Bicep	Bicep curl 15	Bicep curl 15	Bicep curl 15
Tricep	Tricep extension 15	Tricep extension 15	Tricep extension 15
Abs	Ab crunch 20	Ab crunch 20	Ab crunch 20
Forearms	Forearm curl 15	Forearm curl 15	Forearm curl 15

You need to complete your workout and get dressed for that dinner in half an hour. Now is not the time to go through a long-winded routine. Instead, you can couple two exercises in a **combination exercise** and complete your **total body routine** in a matter of 20–30 minutes—all of which are great for fat loss. Essentially, you address more than one muscle group in each exercise.

SOME EXAMPLES OF COMBINATION EXERCISES

Body Parts	Exercise
Shoulders + Glutes + Legs	Military press + Squats
Shoulders + Chest + Legs + Core	Burpees
Glutes + Legs + Arms	Pulse lunges + Bicep curls
Legs + Arms	Calf raises + Overhead tricep extensions
Chest + Shoulders + Legs + Core	Spiderman
Cardio + Glutes + Legs	Lunge walking

Please remember that these are advanced exercises, not to be done by just anybody. For you to be able to perform a combination exercise, you should first be able to perform each individual exercise with perfect form.

When weight training is carried out in the above ways, without a break, using the heaviest weight you can manage with excellent form, the calorie expenditure is at its maximum. It is almost like a cardio. Your heart rate will be elevated, you will be sweating while at the same time toning and sculpting your body. As a result of the elevated intensity the calorie burn continues to remain elevated (however marginally) even after the workout. This allows for fat loss and an elevated basal metabolic rate.

I see women go through their weight training, swinging their weights casually, with no idea whatsoever which muscle they are working or even how to execute the move correctly. Don't waste your time! If you want to train with weights, do so correctly. I am also reluctant to subscribe to the new trend of working with weights to music as part of your cardio class. The last few minutes are spent swinging a couple of light dumb-bells around. I believe weight training needs to have a different focus from cardio—the whole mindset is different. One needs to be taught weight training, muscle names and exercises to be able to understand what one is doing with those weights. Of course, weights can be done to music, at a much slower tempo, however, and with the sole focus on the muscle being worked.

Questions & DIY

- How many times a week do you train with weights?
- Are you now able to identify your muscles and the exercises that train them?
- What is the weight (in kg or lb) you use for:
  Chest press:
  Rowing:
  Shoulder press:
  Bicep curls:
  Tricep extensions:
  Squats:
- How many push-ups can you do with proper form?

- How many sit-ups can you do with proper form?

- Why do you think you need to train with weights?

Strength Training Quick Facts

- Strength training is an **absolutely essential, non-negotiable** aspect of fitness for women.
- There are several **misconceptions about weight training**, particularly pertaining to women, that have hopefully been clarified in this chapter.
- **Benefits of strength training** go beyond aesthetics, to improved balance, posture, bone mass, metabolism, self-confidence, and so on.
- Before you start training, set your goals. What are you hoping to achieve? More muscle mass? Greater strength or endurance? Your prescription for weight training should vary accordingly.

- Perform 4-6 sets of 6-12 reps (70 per cent intensity) for muscular strength; 3 sets of 15-20 reps for muscle endurance; and 5-8 sets of 6-8 reps for size of the muscle.
- Some **basic principles**, like breathing, positioning of the knees and other joints, and protecting the back, need to be followed meticulously while weight-training. Never compromise on these principles in the hope of achieving faster or better results. All you will incur is injury.
- Training effectively, even **twice a week** is sufficient to see results.
- Learn to identify which body part and which muscles you are working with, in each exercise. That way you know where you need to feel the effort of the exercise, and are less likely to injure yourself.
- Over a period of time, you should be able to **train independently** and follow any routine given to you. That is how well you need to know your exercises.
- **Rest** and **nutrition** play an important role in weight training.
- **Supplements** like protein, amino acids and creatine are not mandatory, and excellent results can be achieved without subjecting yourself to these additions if proper training routines are followed.
- Work with your body, not against it. If you are inherently a small-built individual, with a small frame and little muscle mass, building enormous proportions will be a Herculean task (not impossible but Herculean). Keep that in mind and decide if you are prepared for the challenge. Aim instead to build adequate muscle to keep you looking toned and lean.
- In order to achieve muscle definition, you need to **lose the fat over the muscle**. Cardio and diet are an essential aspect of getting that lean, sculpted look.
- Strategies like super-setting, circuit training and combination exercises save time and **increase fat burn**.

CHAPTER 7

PILLAR 3

MUSCLE ENDURANCE

Muscle endurance is closely related to your stamina, but is not really the same thing. Endurance is also very different from the strength of the muscle. Have you ever experienced a situation where you are breathing comfortably, not winded during your workout, but after a while your leg muscles cramp and you need to sit down and rest them? Alternatively, on a long Sunday walk, have you felt your legs tire after a couple of hours of walking comfortably, even though you are not breathless?

What is happening here is that your heart and lungs (your stamina) are adequate and not really being challenged, but the muscle endurance of your legs is not up to specs. The reverse may also hold true. Your leg muscles may be fine but you are so breathless that you need to stop.

SLOW TWITCH AND FAST TWITCH FIBRES

The two types of muscle fibres in our body function differently. The slow twitch fibres, otherwise called Type 1 fibres, can continue to work for prolonged periods of time, but cannot exert too much force. They are efficient at using oxygen as fuel and generating energy in the form of ATP (adenosine triphosphate). The fast twitch fibres, on the other hand, can exert a tremendous amount of force but can only work for short periods of time. They are more efficient in generating ATP in the anaerobic metabolic pathway. Slow twitch fibres are essential for long-duration endurance activities like marathons, whereas the fast twitch fibres are more important for strength, power and short bursts of intense activity like sprinting. We are concerned here solely with developing endurance of muscle. Examples of activities using slow twitch fibres which develop endurance are:

- Long-distance running like marathons and cross-country running
- Triathlons
- Long-distance biking, swimming
- Cross-country skiing.

To improve endurance, long-duration exercises are:

- Slow long walks or runs
- Climbing hundreds of stairs slowly to work your muscles, not test your stamina
- A step workout done slowly to test leg muscle endurance
- Long, slow bike rides
- Rowing or ergometer to improve upper body endurance
- Doing 25 reps of the same exercise in one set.

It is a good idea to intersperse intense activities like a HIIT session, heavy weight-training sessions or boot camp with one or two slower longer-endurance activities during the course of the week. It balances out the body and prevents overtraining. On the other hand, solely engaging in endurance training like walking for an hour or two every day, as I see many people do, will lead to muscle depletion. This has to be counteracted with strength training if you want to maintain muscle mass.

TOUR DE FRANCE

The Tour is probably one of the finest examples of the test of muscle endurance and stamina. The cyclists cover 2,162 miles over 21 days. Rough terrain and uncertain weather can make it one of the most gruelling sports ever. My fascination for the sport brought about an even greater sense of respect and awe for the enormous capabilities of the human body. How many of us can actually say we challenge it, respect it and nourish it the way we are supposed to?

CHAPTER 8

PILLAR 4

FLEXIBILITY

I see people rushing through their workout routines with a few cursory stretches, mainly to appease the trainer, usually in a hurry to get going. Their flexibility does not get any better; they can still barely bend forward to reach for their knees leave alone their toes, but they see no reason in wasting time toiling with stretches. They figure, they have more important things to do.

One could not be more mistaken. An inflexible muscle is not half as strong as it appears to be, whatever the size or shape. It is more prone to injury and cannot perform as well as it should. Good quality muscle is supple, strong and flexible. Flexibility is the cornerstone of fitness along with stamina and strength. For some reason, however, it has always been treated with some disdain, considered an annoying waste of time.

The effects of improved flexibility, however, are subtle and enviable—better posture, greater and more fluid mobility, grace of movement, symmetry and aesthetics. Stretching to improve flexibility is the process by which one's muscles are elongated to their optimum in order to keep them supple. Muscles are elastic and can be stretched. They respond well to a progressive stretching and strengthening programme, making them better balanced and stronger.

FORMS OF STRETCHING

Dynamic stretching   Static stretching

Dynamic stretching: Begin your workout with a few dynamic stretches. Dynamic stretching combines the slow and repeated movement of muscles along with a stretch that helps warm them up. This type of stretching has gained momentum now in sports circles. It reduces the risk of injury in runners, soccer players and recreational exercisers. It is performed by propelling the muscles to their maximum range of motion. The motion has to be smooth and controlled, not jerky or abrupt. The movement is repeated 10-20 times until the concerned muscles are warm and stretched. Some examples of dynamic stretches are alternate knee lifts, butt kicks, side lunges, forward lunges and torso twists. Yoga sequences like the Sun Salutation or Surya Namaskar can also be used as a dynamic stretch. Doing about 6-12 Sun Salutations in quick succession before a workout stretches and warms up practically all the major muscles in the body.

This is what we practise at TFL. The students are taught the Sun Salutation, are corrected innumerable times until they get it right, and are encouraged to progress with it. The Sun Salutation calls for strength, balance and flexibility. It can be modified for a beginner and adapted to suit a more advanced exerciser. We use it as a warm-up even before a regular weight-training session.

Static stretching is accomplished with the body in a stationary position or when the body is at rest. The muscle that needs to be stretched is usually assisted by other parts of the body and stretched to the point of mild discomfort, not pain. Each stretch is usually held for about 20-30 seconds.

A static stretch routine is excellent when done at the end of an exercise routine after the muscles have warmed up. It releases the tension in the muscles, produces a feeling of relaxation and helps you unwind after a strenuous routine. The static stretch should not be done prior to a warm-up. Stretching a cold muscle can lead to injury. Runners who routinely perform static, quad, calf and hamstring stretches before their run, but after a sufficient warm-up, were found to have a lower performance than those who performed dynamic stretches.

The illustration in the following pages is a 3-minute stretch. It addresses all the muscles of the body and can be done anywhere, even in the midst of a long workday. Each stretch is held for about 20 seconds.

FOR HOW LONG TO STRETCH?

A muscle takes about 6-12 seconds to even begin to stretch. Holding the stretched position in a static stretch for about **20-30 seconds**, therefore, should suffice to maintain flexibility. **The stretch cycle needs to be repeated 2-3 times.** However, if you want to improve the flexibility of a certain muscle you would need to hold the position for about a minute, repeating the cycle 2-3 times. In yoga, most poses are held for about a minute to maximize the stretch of the corresponding body part.

3-Minute Stretch

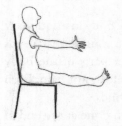

Foot and Hand
Stretch

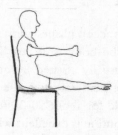

Foot and Hand
Squeeze

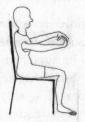

Forearm Stretch
(Repeat on Both
Hands)

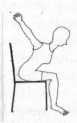

Chest Stretch

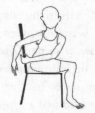

Spinal Twist
(Repeat on Both
Sides)

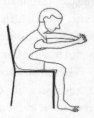

Back Stretch

Neck Stretch

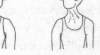

Neck Stretch

3-Minute Stretch

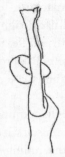

Side and Upper Back Stretch

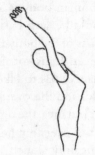

Chest and Side Stretch

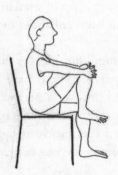

Glute Stretch
(Repeat on Both Sides)

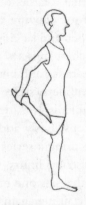

Quad Stretch
(Repeat on Both Sides)

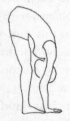

Hamstring and Low Back Stretch

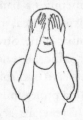

Rest the Eyes and Relax

MUSCLE IMBALANCE

The human body is a beautifully engineered machine. Ideally it should be well balanced with the front and back, right and left parts of the body being equal in size, strength and flexibility. However, this is not always the case. The management of muscle imbalances has to take into account the inflexibility of certain muscles and the overstretched antagonists.

For instance, the tight, obstinate chest muscles in conjunction with the overstretched and weak upper back muscles lead to the ungainly slouch of the upper back, and the rolling in of the shoulders—the 'head and neck forward syndrome'. If the internal rotators of the shoulders are tighter than the external rotators, drawing the shoulders inward causes one to appear stooped and lacking in confidence. The simple act of stretching the chest muscles and strengthening the back enhances one's appearance and bearing.

Runners suffer from tight hamstrings, hip flexors and pyriformis (the deep muscles of the pelvis). These have to be consciously and meticulously worked on over a period of time using a series of stretches in order to improve their run. Hamstring injury is also common when the muscle is tight, and this sets one back several months before one can get back into training again.

Not all injuries are due to tight or inflexible muscles, however. Sometimes a hamstring injury in a runner could be the result of weak gluteal muscles, an unstable pelvis or problems with the lumbar spine. Stretching the hamstrings alone, in this case, will not suffice. Strengthening of the gluteal muscles and stabilizing the pelvis and spine will be required. It is important to consult with a professional to deal holistically with the problem.

If you are accustomed to repeating a particular kind of activity all the time such as the stepping action in the step class, climbing uphill in incline-walking, or the kicking and punching action in a kick-boxing class, you can be sure of developing muscle imbalances unless these are checked early with stretching and strengthening routines. **This is a form of repetitive stress injury or RSI.**

So what do you do? Don't relegate flexibility to the back-burner and promise yourself you will stretch over the weekend. It has to be done every day. Allot a couple of days a week for a longer, more extensive stretch routine. Over a period of time your flexibility will improve. You will be consciously better balanced and have a more elegant posture.

Don't stretch cold muscles. Have you ever watched children play with Play-Doh? Cold Play-Doh is not malleable and is difficult to mould. As the child works with it and warms it up, pummelling and pushing it, it gives and becomes more supple. It is the same with our muscles. They need to be slightly warm to be capable of stretching. Forcing a cold muscle to stretch will only injure it.

Perform some dynamic stretches before your workout. Avoid bouncing (ballistic) movements while stretching. A dynamic stretch is a smooth flowing motion taken to its completion and repeated several times. Proceed with the rest of the workout and follow up with extensive static stretches after your workout.

Each muscle can be stretched using a particular movement. It is worth learning these exercises and ensuring that they are done properly to avoid injury with overstretching. Assisted stretches with a trainer or partner need to be performed with caution as sometimes the partner has no way of determining how much is too much for you and may inadvertently injure the muscle.

Ageing muscle: One of the most important benefits of regular stretching is the capacity to remain flexible with age. Certain muscles like the hamstrings and low back muscles tend to become tight, and often lead to backache and discomfort that so commonly plagues older people. As one ages, muscles become less elastic. This inflexibility can lead to difficulty in performing simple tasks like turning to reverse the car or reaching for that bottle of spices at the back of the overhead cupboard. Continuing to stretch daily will prevent this unfortunate turn of events, keeping you independent, self-confident and agile.

Yoga is an excellent addition to your fitness routine. The practice of yoga is often presented in twenty-first-century marketing terms as the ultimate beauty tool. It now enjoys the endorsement of conventional medicine.

Yoga can be adapted for an individual just like any other form of exercise. You need a good teacher who understands your needs and who is able to teach, motivate and inspire you to grow in your yogic practice. Yoga can be used as a supplement and complement to your cardio and weight training. It does not have to be exclusive of other aspects of your fitness routine. We use the Sun Salutation as part of our warm-up before weight training and cardio, or as a stretch after a workout. We teach several yoga routines (vinyasas) that may be practised to primarily improve flexibility but also strength and balance. They are beautiful when done well, and extremely effective.

> Payal had delivered a beautiful baby boy in May. By September, she had lost all her pregnancy fat; but she was unhappy about one thing. Her shoulders rolled in, making her seem hunched, shorter, lacking in confidence and tired.
>
> 'What is wrong with my body?' she asked almost in tears. 'I am back to my pre-pregnancy weight but I look different, shorter and heavier.'

The weight of her breasts and breastfeeding the baby were creating the rolled-in shoulders. We had to work on many corrections and realign the upper body.

Payal was started on:

- Strengthening exercises for the **upper back and shoulders**.
- She was then given **progressive stretching and strengthening** for the chest muscles and upper arms. In addition, she worked on the deep rotator cuff muscles of the shoulders and the rhomboids (the muscles between the shoulder blades), which drew her shoulders back and opened up her chest.
- She was made to do **lateral angle series** 3 times a week to open up the chest, strengthen the legs, improve flexibility in the legs, and improve her balance and core strength.
- Within 2 weeks of strengthening and stretching she began to look taller and regained her original elegance, which, somehow in the midst of nappy changing and feeding, had sunk in along with her shoulders.

She is back to training regularly now to keep up with the demands of new motherhood. We focused primarily on strength training for her at that point, the cardio kept to the minimum of 20 minutes a day. She trained seriously to build strength and muscle in her legs and upper body, and focused on stabilizing and strengthening her core, as pregnancy invariably takes its toll on the core muscles.

Questions & DIY

1. Do you do static stretches or dynamic stretches, and when do you do them?

2. Are you aware of which muscle you are stretching? Is your focus on the muscle being stretched?

3. How long do you hold each static stretch?

4.   Seated with legs extended, can you reach your toes and touch your forehead to your knees (hamstring and low back stretch)?

5.   Standing erect, can you bend forward and touch the floor with your palms without bending the knees?

6.   Do you enjoy stretching? Does it relax you?

7.   Do you try to improve the degree of your stretches and reach further each time?

8.   Did you know there are specific stretches for different sports?

9.   Did you know muscle imbalance, injury and bad posture can be corrected and prevented with an appropriate stretching routine?

10. Did you know that when you are very exhausted and unable to do a cardio and weight-training routine, you could do a 5-minute dynamic stretch to warm the muscles and then follow up with a slow 20-minute stretch routine, and feel fantastic afterwards?

CHAPTER 9

NUTRITION

FOOD FOR THOUGHT

Dear Diet,

I just don't think it's going to work out between us. It's over between you and me. You are boring, tasteless and I can't stop cheating on you!

Sincerely,

Me

Understanding your food and not considering it an adversary is critical if you want to spend your days enjoying the innumerable options for the palate, while at the same time maintaining your weight at a healthy optimum. The word diet conjures up images of cabbage soup, celery sticks and near starvation. It does not have to be this way! In fact, starving yourself into your new dress will only lead to a lowered basal metabolic rate (BMR), as the body perceives a famine around the corner. This sluggish metabolism does you no good when you get back to eating even near normal food, at which point you find, to your disgust, that you have begun to gain all the weight you've lost and more.

When you decide to go on a diet, ask yourself these questions:

- Is it **balanced**? Does it provide you with not just energy (plain white sugar can do that), but nutrition for your body, your skin, nails and hair?

- Is it **sustainable**? If it is something you can just about manage to continue for about a week or a couple of days, chances are that it will not be of great benefit in the long term. After the diet is over, in all likelihood, you will go back to eating senselessly.

- Does it allow you to eat from **all the food groups** and in moderation? Does it restrict the intake of refined carbohydrates like refined white rice, flour and sugar? Does it allow you instead to consume whole unrefined foods including fruits and vegetables which also belong to the carbohydrate group?

- Severe restrictions from specific food groups, such as no carbs or zero fat, only serve to stimulate cravings over time, not to mention nutritional deficiencies. A balanced diet allows you to eat from all the groups, but in moderation. Once you are educated about your choices, you will learn to implement them cleverly.

- Is it **laborious and time-consuming** to fulfil all the prerequisites of the diet? For instance, does the diet insist you drink strange concoctions, eat only specific combinations of food, spend all your time cooking intricate recipes so you find yourself obsessing about your food, your menu and your diet all day?

- Does it require you to eat **specific branded products**?

Chances are, it is the company making the products that will benefit more than you.

Why is it that our body invariably steers itself towards fattening foods? Perhaps it is the sense of satisfaction that fat provides, the sheer decadence. One has to keep in mind that fat provides 9 calories/gram. Both carbohydrates and protein, on the other hand, provide only 4 calories/gram. The **overconsumption of fats** can increase your total calorie intake enormously, and cause weight gain. Not to say that the overconsumption of other food groups is harmless.

Over time, with improved awareness about food and nutrition, you learn to identify that there are different kinds of carbohydrates, proteins and fats, some of which are essentially good for you and which your body needs. **You stop obsessing about just calorific values and focus instead on the quality of calories.** You can get about 200 calories from an oil-ridden paratha made totally from refined white flour. You can also get 200 calories from a smaller-sized wholewheat paratha with a little peanut oil and stuffed with grated radish. So, which is better? You can make that decision without too much uncertainty.

We not only have to nourish our bodies with food, but also enjoy the food and celebrate it. This does not mean we eat indiscriminately, but that we eat good, nutritious and tasty food to satisfy all our senses—taste, smell, sight and, of course, hunger. Depriving our body of food and nutrition will eventually lead to its detriment.

Unless you understand your food, you will be on an eternal quest for that magic diet that you believe will get you to miraculously shed kilos. High protein? Low carb? High fat? Low fat?—the various diets available to us are awe-inspiring but confusing.

I notice that when I explain the food pyramid and a balanced diet to some women, they are just not impressed!

'So what you are telling me is that I have to eat all these things, the red rice, vegetables, dal, fruit and eggs. But then how can that be a diet?' Sonali weighed 90 kg. She had been struggling with her weight all her life. She had sampled every diet possible on the planet, including some strange ones I had never heard of. What amazed me was that despite her obvious lack of success with these diets, she was still hopeful that there was this elusive one she had missed in her quest, which would help her achieve her weight loss goal.

'Sonali, there is no magic diet to burn the fat,' I tried to explain. 'It's about eating balanced healthy food as a lifestyle.'

'You mean all my life?' She looked unbelieving and was almost in tears. 'How is that possible? It's too simple. Not possible.'

Like Sonali, to many women diet means:
- A complicated combination of foods that promise to burn fat,
- Food restrictions that guarantee inch loss,
- Foods to be consumed at specific times that assure you of slimmer thighs.

The fact of the matter is that the food pyramid is the only way to **make a healthy, balanced diet a lifestyle**. Consuming all food groups in sufficient quantities and proper portions will ensure weight loss in a healthy, manageable way. It is also the only diet you can sustain without getting deprived of essential nutrients. Most importantly, you have a fair amount of control over it without being instructed or directed by someone else.

You have to first ascertain how many calories you require in a day. This depends on your activity level, weight, gender, and whether you need to lose fat, gain muscle or maintain your weight. Then determine how many servings you need from each of the food groups in the food pyramid. Then plan your diet.

THE FOOD PYRAMID

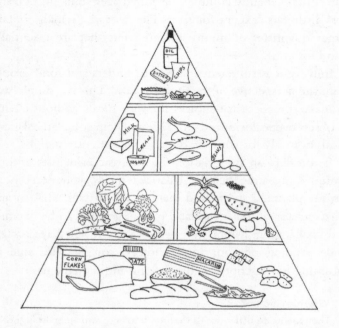

Your body needs all the food groups. Singling out one to eat to the exclusion of others could send you into a tailspin of deficiencies and cravings. A well-balanced diet, with the right combination of carbohydrates, proteins, fats, micronutrients, minerals and vitamins, combining all the food groups, is absolutely essential to sustain health and a positive frame of mind.

Most of the food groups contain a combination of nutrients. The foods under bread/cereal for instance, besides containing carbohydrates, will also have varying amounts of protein, some fats, minerals and vitamins. Vegetables and fruits also contain, mainly, complex carbohydrates, some protein and very little fats (except for fruits like avocado, which contain larger quantities of mono-saturated fats that are essentially good for you).

Initially, it is sufficient for you to understand food groups from the perspective of the food pyramid. This is a simple way to make the necessary choices for your meals without having to obsess over calories and fats. This will help you plan balanced meals not only for yourself, but also for the entire family.

If you have an appreciation for the basic principles of food groups and eating healthy, balanced meals, you don't need anyone planning specialized diets or telling you what to and what not to eat. Balancing and planning food can be exciting and challenging. Menus can get creative. If you have a clear understanding of your food choices, you will be able to substitute healthy options for cooking and ingredients.

Who are calories?
They are nasty little rascals that get into your wardrobe at night and shrink your clothes!

—*Anon.*

THE BREAD/CEREAL GROUP

Each gram of carbohydrates provides 4 calories. In India, we tend to consume way too much of the cereal/grain faction and way too little of the fruits and vegetables, which we nearly kill and then try to resuscitate with our methods of cooking. This was probably, originally, for economic reasons, rice or wheat being cheaper than vegetables.

What is 1 serving? Any one of the following:

- ½ cup cooked rice
- 1 roti without oil (about 15 cm in diameter)
- ½ cup cooked oats
- 1 cup dry cereal like cornflakes
- 1 idli/dosa
- 1 slice wholewheat bread

A small cup, which amounts to 2 servings of cooked rice or 2 slices of wholewheat bread, should suffice for one meal for most women. When eaten with adequate amounts of vegetables, protein in the form of lentils or the meat protein (as long as it is not drowning in a soup of oil), it should satisfy you.

Most women would need about 5 servings of the bread/cereal group in an entire day. Do the math; with an Indian diet, that would include:

- 2 idlis *or* 1 cup poha *or* 1 cup cooked oatmeal for breakfast
- ½ cup cooked rice for lunch
- 2 small rotis for dinner

Please note, this is an example for a woman who requires about 1400 cal/day. Not everyone does, some may require more and some even less.

For an Indian woman this may come as a shock.

'How can I survive on such meagre quantities of rice, rotis?'

Well, that's all you really need! When the necessary supplements, like lentils, vegetables, fruit and yogurt, are included in the meal it should more than suffice.

'But if 1 serving of the bread/cereal group has just 80 calories (approximately) why can't I have more?'

Here's the problem. It doesn't stop with just the extra serving of the bread/cereal group, does it? One has to accompany the rice with some gravy (usually oily), a couple of pieces of meat,

more pickle, some fried chips perhaps...the list is endless, and
the final result is an unacceptable accumulation of consumed
calories. In addition, eating more from this food group will
mean you eat less from the others, or will not include all the
other groups.

If you restrict yourself to the required number of servings
in ALL the food groups, however, you will find yourself sated
and nourished.

THE FRUIT AND VEGETABLE GROUP

Fruits and vegetables also come under the general umbrella
of carbohydrates. Vegetables (except potato, yam, pea, corn,
tapioca and sweet potato, which come under the bread/cereal
group) are particularly low in calories and very filling at the
same time—a great reason to include a salad with every meal.
A minimum of 2-3 fruits and 3-4 servings of vegetables per day
on an average is required to provide us with all the minerals,
vitamins, phytochemicals and antioxidants.

What is 1 serving? Any one of the following:
- ½ cup vegetable, cooked or raw
- I cup leafy vegetables like spinach or salad leaves
- I average-sized fruit: the size of a tennis ball
- ¾ cup fruit juice
- ¼ cup dried fruit: about 3-4 dates
- ½ cup canned fruit

The greens—spinach, amaranth, methi, and a wide variety
of indigenous greens that are available in our country—are
an excellent source of iron, fibre and numerous minerals and
vitamins. They are extremely low in calories, can be cooked
in various ways and make excellent complements to Indian
meals. Include greens into your menu every day. Low-calorie
vegetables also include the gourd variety, brinjal, lady's finger,

pumpkin, runner bean, string bean, capsicum, colocasia, tomato, cucumber, cabbage, cauliflower and Brussels sprout.

Most women I counsel don't consume enough of fruits and vegetables. The veggies are placed in the far corner of the plate and eaten grudgingly. Worse, they are sometimes overcooked, mangled, disfigured, and smothered in various oils until their very flavour is lost. We do have several delicious vegetarian dishes in our country. Many of them are also highly nutritious, if cooked with less oil. With the current trend in obesity, I do not think we can afford to eat dishes immersed in oil all the time.

Veggie soups are a great way to curtail hunger while obtaining a wide variety of micronutrients. Make them clear or with a purée of vegetables as the base instead of thickening with cornflour or cream.

A mention here of the mighty potato that has evoked such conflict with the low carb, no carb craze. The potato is highly nutritious but also high in starch. It needs to be viewed not as a vegetable but as part of the bread/cereal group. The equivalent of 1 serving of bread/cereal for the potato would be 1 medium-sized potato. When viewed from this perspective, it can feature as a part of your menu, when positioned in its appropriate place.

Similarly, corn is part of the bread/cereal group. Half a cup of corn kernels being the equivalent of 1 serving.

I do think, as Indians, we eat too many refined carbs at the expense of vegetables, fruits and nuts. Take a masala dosa or aloo puri—carbs and more carbs! Where is the protein? In the tiny speck of watered-down sambar you tentatively dipped the dosa in? Lunch for an Indian could easily mean 3-4 cups of a variety of rices (delicious, no doubt!) with potatoes, tapioca or a few vegetables, maybe a couple of pieces of fried fish. Can we keep those servings of refined carbs down? I am not saying don't ever eat a masala dosa or aloo puri. Just understand where it fits into the whole scheme of the food pyramid and restrict such indulgences to an occasion.

Fibre is a form of complex carbohydrate. A high-fibre diet gives the feeling of satiety without the added calories. Fibre is present mainly in roots, skins, leaves and seeds. Processing or refining foods removes the fibre. In our diet, the main sources of fibre are whole unrefined grains, whole fruits, vegetables, legumes, nuts and seeds. Fibre is important not only for satiety but also for protection against heart disease and to keep the digestive system healthy. Constipation, haemorrhoids, gall bladder disease and diverticulitis are all common when fibre in the food is restricted. The recommended amount of fibre intake is about 25-30 gm/day. Soluble fibre, found in oats, barley, fruits and legumes, has been found to bind and excrete fats from the body—one reason why they are known to lower cholesterol levels and blood sugar. Insoluble fibre, found in skins and roots, wholewheat and cereals, absorbs water in the intestines, forming softer, bulkier stool for easier evacuation. Insoluble fibre has also been found to bind to carcinogens, lowering the risk of colon cancer.

As with everything, more fibre is not better, however. Too much fibre can cause loss of phosphorus, calcium and iron and gastrointestinal discomfort.

The Glycemic Index (GI) is a way of ranking carbohydrate foods based on how quickly they are absorbed into the system to increase blood sugar levels.
   Low GI foods are:
* Those that are higher in fibre and absorbed more slowly,
* Lead to a slower increase in blood sugar levels.

- Especially important for people with diabetes to keep blood sugar on an even keel and avoid sudden spiking.
- Examples of low GI foods are oats, wholewheat, whole grains like rye, barley, millet, red rice and ragi.

High GI foods are:

- usually refined foods that are absorbed quickly causing a sudden and rapid spike in the blood sugar followed by an immediate elevation of insulin.
- These include refined carbs like refined flour, sugar, white rice and white bread.

Focusing on unrefined, high-fibre, wholegrain cereals and minimizing rapidly absorbed, refined cereals and sugary foods will all help to lower the GI of your diet. Eating mainly low GI foods ensures that you maintain your blood sugar and insulin levels on an even keel. This is important from a weight perspective also. **Sudden spikes of blood insulin have been found to favour fat accumulation leading to obesity.** Sweetened fruit juices, sweetened cereals, refined grains, cakes, cookies, biscuits, packaged salted fried snacks, and sweetened alcoholic drinks are the usual offenders. These foods are not only tasty but also extremely addictive, easy to access but disastrous for the waistline.

'It takes all my will power not to be tempted by the chips, salted fried nuts and various packaged foods in the house, Doctor.' Christine sounded very self-righteous.

'But why do you stock them?' I asked.

She looked at me as if I had asked her an obviously self-explanatory question. 'Why, of course I have to. My kids come home from school starving and they simply have to eat something immediately. My husband needs his snacks with his drink at night. So you see, my hands are tied really. What to do!'

This is a common excuse I hear all the time. The kids need it? The husband needs it? Do they really? If it is not good for you, how can it be good for them?

'Oh, they get very upset if they don't have their favourite snacks.'

A majority of the women in our country have the responsibility of making decisions in the kitchen. There may be preferences from in-laws, children and the husband. By and large, however, a smart woman should learn how to substitute healthy, tasty options for stupid ones. It will of course require thought, planning and definitely more work than buying a packet of chips from the store down the road. Nevertheless, it is well worth the effort if you consider the health of your family.

Make a list of healthy snacks you and your kids can eat when they come back from school. A snack should ideally contain foods from both the carb group and the protein group for slower absorption and longer satiety.

a. 2 slices of French toast with wholewheat bread and eggs.

b. 2 slices of cheese toast with wholewheat bread.

c. Bhel puri with grated vegetables, mint and tomato chutney. Garnished with puffed rice, chopped coriander, mango, onions, tomato and a handful of nuts.

d. 1 cup of soy upma with plenty of veggies.

e. 2½ eggs omelette (1 whole egg and 3 egg whites) with plenty of veggies, mushrooms and a slice of cheese.

f. A wholewheat-and-soy-rotis wrap with lettuce, cucumber, tomato and avocado.

g. A handful of roasted nuts.

h. 1 whole cob of corn.

i. Strawberry yogurt smoothie with 1 tsp honey and 3-4 walnut halves.

j. Broken wheat and lentils steamed and stir-fried with 1 cup of grated carrot, beans and peas.

Making Sense of the Carbs

- The **bread/cereal group** (grains, rice, rotis, idlis, kakras, upma, poha, oats and cornflakes), the **vegetable group** and the **fruit group** contain mainly carbs.
- Carbs are necessary as a quick source of energy and nutrients, and should not be eliminated completely from your diet.
- Consume more vegetables and fruits and keep **the bread/ cereal** to **the absolute minimum** number of servings depending on your weight and activity level—4-5 servings if you are not active, 7-8 if you are **very** active.
- Eat 3 different coloured vegetables every day.
- Eat 2 different fruits every day. Whole fruits are better than the juices.
- On your plate, only a quarter of the plate needs to be filled with your bread/cereal option.
- The total number of servings of the bread/cereal you consume in a day should be within the number you are allowed and preferably spread out during the course of the day. However, if you do consume most of your **bread/cereal** options in one meal, the rest of your meals should contain only the other options—the vegetables, fruit, protein and milk groups.
- A plate of delicious biryani, the timeless Indian delicacy, can consist of all 5 servings of your bread/cereal option for the day. So you can now figure out what you should be eating the rest of the day...

THE PROTEIN GROUP

Every gram of protein provides 4 calories. Protein is present in meat, poultry, fish, eggs, beans, nuts and soy products. These foods also contain a fair amount of fats. Red meats particularly tend to have a higher percentage of saturated fat. Keeping red meat to the minimum and focusing on oily fish and poultry is a healthier option.

The vegetarian sources are lentils, beans, soy and nuts. The various grains like amaranth, quinoa and millet also contain a higher percentage of protein than rice. Obtaining sufficient protein while on a vegetarian, or even a vegan, diet is not impossible but requires some thought and understanding of which foods to include. Quinoa has been touted as a wonder grain. It contains a very high percentage of protein for a grain. It is not readily available in India, however.

Most vegetarian sources of protein are considered incomplete proteins as they do not contain all the essential amino acids that are required for the body. However, classic food combinations like red rice and kidney beans can balance the protein requirements.

A vegetarian, especially a vegan, would require the vitamin B12 supplement, however, as this vitamin is not found in plant foods and a deficiency can cause anaemia and nerve damage.

The **protein requirement** has been evaluated to be 0.8 gm of protein/kg body weight for an adult, 1 gm/kg if you are weight-training. Protein is required for muscle-building and repair of tissues. But, on consumption, it does not go directly to the muscle and enable it to grow. You have to work out for that! Overdosing on protein is quite possible and certainly not beneficial.

Isolated amino acids have really not been found to be more beneficial than whole proteins in food. These supplements are expensive and need to be monitored. You also need to work out accordingly to compensate for the intake.

A woman weighing 55 kg who is training regularly will require 55 x 1 = 55 gm of protein in a day. Higher amounts of protein are required for professional bodybuilders.

What is 1 serving?

Non-vegetarian options: 1 serving is the equivalent of about 85 gm of any of the following:

- Chicken: 1 chicken breast grilled/roasted
- Mutton/Beef: 3-4 pieces, the size of a deck of cards
- Fish: 1 mackerel, or 1½ slice of seerfish
- Eggs: 3

Vegetarian options: 1 serving is the equivalent of 85 gm of any of the following:

- Cooked lentils: 1½ cups
- Soy: 1½ cups
- Nuts: ¾ cup

If you are allowed 140 gm of protein, for instance, you could divide it up into 1 egg (28 gm), 1 cup lentils (56 gm), ¼ cup nuts (28 gm), ½ cup soy (28 gm).

THE MILK GROUP

What is 1 serving? Any of the following:

- 1 cup milk (226 gm)
- 1 cup yogurt
- 1 oz cheese (28 gm)

An average woman requiring 1400 cal/day will need 2 servings from the milk group. Keep the calorie intake limited by restricting yourself to low fat milk and yogurt. Don't forget to include the milk you add to the numerous cups of tea and coffee in a day when you recall your diet.

Pregnant women, breastfeeding mothers and younger children need 3 servings of the milk group. It can be in the form of yogurt, a smoothie with fruits, or cheese. I know mothers who wail about their 5-year-olds hating milk. Get innovative. Make him a strawberry smoothie.

FATS

Each gram of fat provides 9 calories. Fats are present naturally in various foods. Even grains contain some amount of fats. Some foods, like nuts, seeds, red meats and high fat dairy products like cheese, are obviously higher in fat content than fibrous vegetables like greens and broccoli, and fruits like citrus fruits, pears and apples. We also use fats in the form of oils, ghee and butter as a medium for cooking to add flavour to food. *Half a litre of oil per adult per month is more than sufficient for cooking purposes. Approximately 5-6 tsp of oil per individual per day.*

Saturated fats are those present in animal products such as meat, milk, butter, ghee and ice cream. These fats are usually solid at room temperature. They have been found to raise blood cholesterol levels which cause coronary heart disease and blocked vessels.

Unsaturated fats are those derived from vegetable sources. Oils derived from canola, sesame, linseed, olives, peanuts and walnuts are called monounsaturated fatty acids or **MUFA**. Avocados contain a high percentage of monounsaturated fats that are essentially good for you. Oils derived from corn, sunflower, soybean and sesame contain polyunsaturated fatty acids or **PUFA**. Polyunsaturated oils like sunflower have been popularized as the solution to high cholesterol. However, consuming solely this form of oil can be detrimental to health. Switch between groundnut oil, sesame oil, sunflower oil, olive oil, rice bran oil, almond oil and linseed oil. The different oils may be used in different cooking methods.

The fatty acids omega-6 and omega-3 are essential for the body and need to be consumed as they cannot be produced by the body itself. Omega-6 fatty acids are found readily in corn and sunflower oil. Omega-3 is found in flaxseed oil, walnuts, soybeans, tofu and certain fish like sardines, mackerel, salmon and tuna. The vegetarian sources of omega-3 are only flaxseeds and walnuts.

Trans Fats

Trans fats are derived when hydrogen is added to liquid vegetable oil. It is also seen in certain forms of animal fat. Hydrogenated oil is used in commercially baked goods like pastries, biscuits and cookies that require a long shelf life. Discrimination against butter led to the development of margarine which contains trans fats. A food containing no animal product may be labelled 'cholesterol free', which may be tempting to buy. Scan the nutritional information carefully. If it contains hydrogenated oils (trans fats) it cannot be good for you. Oil that is reheated several times also contains trans fats. **The problem with trans fats** is that they lead to an elevation of the LDL or bad cholesterol, a lowering of the HDL or good cholesterol and even an increase in triglycerides, basically setting the stage for heart disease. So the next time you buy cream cookies or samosas from the chaatwala, whose wok of oil is always simmering, churning out those delicious crispy treats, you might want to think twice.

Gary Taubes, author of *Good Calories, Bad Calories* and *Why We Get Fat*, believes that fats are not the cause of obesity or responsible for raised cholesterol levels. This is not a new notion; the Atkins diet claimed the same thing. Some believe that saturated fats have been unfairly blamed for heart disease. The contention is that carbohydrates are the real cause of obesity.

Of course, fats cannot be singled out as the cause of obesity.

It is about balanced eating. You do require fats in your diet. They are essential for the working of the cells of the human body, for your skin, the hormones circulating in the body, for the fat-soluble vitamins and digestive system, and for the sense of satisfaction they provide. The problem is that they are present extensively and in unhealthy forms (as trans fats) in various foods, and are sometimes consumed indiscriminately. A tablespoon of peanut butter made with the best quality oil and peanuts contains as much fat as, let's say, a couple of pieces of deep-fried, white flour-encrusted cauliflower fritters, but is obviously better than the latter. Why? It is more nutritious for the same calorie count, and it takes into account the quality of fat used.

Making Sense of Fats

- Fats are present in various foods like oils, butter, ghee, cheese and chocolate, but also in varying quantities in nuts, dairy products, meats and even grains.
- All fat is not bad. The body requires fat for essential functions.
- You do require a minimum amount of fat in your food—20-30 per cent of your daily calorie intake can come from fat.
- Use different types of cooking oils for various forms of cooking.
- The total amount of added oil you require is ½ a litre per adult per month.
- Approximately 5 tsp of oil per individual per day.
- Restrict the sweets, chocolates and deep-fried food to once a week only.
- Avoid processed food and trans fats.

SMALL STEPS GO A LONG WAY

- **Plan your meals.** Problems arise when you are unprepared and eat whatever is available. You are then at the mercy of your hunger.

- Eat **smaller portions.** One cup of rice (2 servings) will go a long way. The most common problem is huge portions. We tend to eat way too much.

- Eat **more frequently**, but stay within your requirement of the number of servings.

- Keep **healthy snack options** ready in case of acute hunger.

- Eat **slowly**.

- **Chew properly.**

- Drink **water** to stay hydrated. A minimum of 8–10 cups a day. More, when you are training and in hot weather.

- Eat from a **smaller plate**. Psychologically, it feels like you have a lot on your plate.

- Use **cutlery**, you tend to eat less with each mouthful and slower.

- Do not spend large parts of the day in starvation only to be ravenous and eat a heavy meal at the end of it.

- Eat a **variety of foods** to enable the absorption of the various micronutrients that are so important in the proper functioning of our body.

- Eat **mindfully**. Do not eat in front of the idiot box. I have done it myself, mindlessly shovelling food into my mouth, engrossed in some inane show. Before you know it, your plate is empty, you have no idea what you just ate and you feel horribly full!

- Fill your **food journal**. This may seem like a hopeless waste of time. It has been found, however, that just the act of filling your journal diligently makes people more introspective about their food choices and aware of the number of servings. In our country we tend to overdo the bread/cereal group. Evaluating food journals of clients, I find most eat up to 10-18 servings of this group in a day. Foods from this group have also become very refined, depleting them of essential nutrition. Maida parathas may be delicious with the oodles of oil, but they are made from refined flour, depleted of everything except calories. You are better benefitted consuming a wholewheat paratha.

Take a typical **South Indian menu** for the day:

Breakfast: 3-4 idlis + ½ cup sambar or lentils + chutney + coffee.

Lunch: 2-3 cups rice + ½ cup dal + ½ cup vegetables, maybe a piece or two of meat + ½ cup yogurt.

Tea: 1 cup tea, crisps, biscuits, some odd snacks that are invariably deep-fried.

Dinner: 2-4 rotis + ½ cup dal + ½ cup vegetables + 1 fruit (maybe).

There you go, that would amount to almost 12 servings of the bread/cereal group in one day. The protein is limited to maybe 85 gm of vegetables, perhaps a cup a day. Maybe a fruit a day and a cup of milk with the numerous teas and coffees. Instead, take a look at the sample diet at the end of the chapter to figure out how to manage your number of servings.

Make a note: 'brown bread' is not the same as wholewheat bread. Bread made with the usual unhealthy, refined flour can be coloured brown using caramelized sugar. You need to ask for wholewheat bread at your bakery. Better still, make your own wholewheat multigrain bread.

Jamie Oliver won the TED prize for his talk *Teach Every Child about Food*. I agree completely. It is imperative that we do so. This mild English gentleman with his famous lisp passionately tells us about growing our own vegetables and cooking hearty and healthy meals. Now, not everyone has the luxury of their own vegetable garden, but we could pay more attention to the foods we buy from the market.

- Source the best place to buy **good quality vegetables and fruits**.
- Shop a couple of times a week for **fresh vegetables**.
- **Avoid stocking up on processed, tinned food**, because although very convenient, they are mostly high in sodium for preservation.
- Try and **cook fresh food** at least once a day.
- Buy **different coloured vegetables** to gain the benefits of the various nutrients in them.
- Don't be shy to sample new and exotic or indigenous vegetables and fruits.
- With world cuisine becoming so popular, one can experiment with various combinations and even create our own menus and recipes as modifications of the originals.

COOKING AT HOME

I learnt to cook early in life. My mother, being an obstetrician, was away most of the time and we had cooks to cook for us. This allowed me the opportunity to experiment in the kitchen from a very young age. Over the years, I have cooked for friends and family (not always successfully!), but as a result, I have learnt the finer nuances of food like I never would have otherwise.

With experience, I dare say I am a fairly decent cook now. What I lack in technique I make up for in imagination! I can never stick with the recipe, I add my own twist, try a healthier version, add new spices, and so on.

Here are some simple tips to keep everyday food light:

- To thicken gravies, use cooked lentils, tomatoes or onions instead of cream, butter or flour.
- Other alternatives to thicken curries are puréed vegetables like knol-khol and marrow, which are basically tasteless and take on the flavour of the dish.
- Add a mix of soy flour, ragi, ground millet and wholewheat flour while making rotis. It adds a variety of nutrients and fibre.
- Add soy flakes to vegetable dishes to include protein, especially if one does not appreciate soy by itself.
- Make your own multigrain bread quite easily with a mix of all the grains.
- Add cooked kidney beans or sprouts to salads.
- Use a yogurt dressing for salads instead of mayo and cream.
- Make your own yogurt dip with yogurt, garlic paste and cilantro to snack on with vegetable fingers.
- Have a smoothie for breakfast with papaya, yogurt and a few walnuts.
- Use a thick-bottomed iron pan or wok to stir-fry vegetables and don't overcook them.
- Have a soup for dinner with a lentil base and vegetables. It is filling and nutritious while being low on calories.

EATING OUT

Eating out in restaurants or in someone else's home is so common these days that learning how to order and eat sensibly is key to keeping calories in check. I don't think being a social butterfly can be used as an excuse to justify gluttony or lack of understanding of food. If you want to look good in your new designer dress while dining in a fancy restaurant, you had better know what not to eat!

Don'ts	Dos
Order a deep-fried appetizer.	Get steamed/stir-fried ones.
Order creamy curries or deep-fried items (kofta, malai, makhni).	Order clear soup, stir-fried; most restaurants will oblige if you specifically request low oil preparations—steamed, grilled, tandoori, sukha rotis, etc.
Order Dal Makhni.	Instead Tadka Dal has less calories.
Order your nans with butter.	Order nans without butter. They still taste great!
Eat everything in the bread basket.	If you just love those oh-so-melting-in-my-mouth breads, then make that your main course.
Over-order. The tendency is to try to eat it all!	You can always order again, if food is insufficient.
Sample every single item in the buffet.	In fact, buffets are really not the best idea for those watching their size. They are proven disasters for your waistline.
Pile your plate with all the forms of the bread/cereal group just because they are available. You will then need to add the complementary side dishes to go with them, and it never ends.	Taste the side dishes if you must. You don't necessarily have to make a whole course of it by eating every single side dish with a bread, roti, biryani, paratha, etc.
Drink too much alcohol, sweetened beverages or even mocktails. They are loaded with unnecessary, empty calories. Besides, alcohol lowers your inhibitions and allows you to indulge in more food!	Stick with water or restrict yourself to one drink or a glass of red wine, which can in fact be good for you.

Don'ts	Dos
Order a whole dessert.	Share with your friends or family; sometimes even a spoonful is quite satisfying.
Be anxious about offending your hostess by not gorging on every single dish at her table.	If she is interested in your well-being, she will understand your need to restrict your calories/portions.
Go to a restaurant or go out for a meal in a state of pure starvation. You will eat indiscriminately.	Have a small, healthy snack before leaving for dinner, especially if it is anticipated to be late.

If you are a savvy eater, you can enjoy the multitude of culinary options available. It all depends on how you manage your calories. If you over-consume one day, you will have to compensate for the indulgence. **Weight gain does not occur overnight, but a succession of parties with rich food and alcohol will pile on the kilos.** It has been found that people gain up to 2 kilos every holiday. If left unchecked, you can well imagine what the end result will be after a few years!

THE MODERN WOMAN

With more women working, time spent in the kitchen cooking fresh meals is uncommon. Young girls learn at an early age that ordering in and eating out of tins is convenient and saves them a lot of trouble. Living in hostels, or sharing apartments with other young girls as is the trend today encourages this behaviour. They don't necessarily have to learn to cook, let alone learn food groups and serving sizes.

It is worth every woman's time, however, to understand food. I mean really understand it. It is not difficult to memorize the food pyramid, food groups and serving sizes. Initially, one may actually need to measure out food so one is familiar with the serving sizes. After a while it becomes easy to eyeball a plate of food and grasp immediately what it contains, the food groups, serving sizes and nutrient value.

Cooking can be very interesting and therapeutic. Sometimes, after a stressful day at work, just cleaning and cutting vegetables or baking bread is de-stressing. So when you do cook, you should attempt to learn more about the food combinations that benefit you and try new healthy recipes. I believe, women, and men for that matter, should be able to put food together and not be solely dependent on home deliveries and eating out. Simple salads, basic meals are not difficult or time-consuming.

> Approach food with respect and caution, delight and pleasure. Observe yourself—do you use it as a defence mechanism, stress buster or comforter? That is not what it should be.

But Isn't Rice Fattening?

'But, I thought rice was fattening,' was a perplexed query I got from a client when I told her she was allowed to have her 1 cup (2 servings) of red rice for lunch.

'Yes it is, if you eat more than you are supposed to,' I tried to explain. 'Every food can be **fattening** or not depending on how much of it you eat. It's about the total number of calories at the end of the day.'

'I have not touched rice for the last 6 months,' she told me rather smugly. 'I was told it was fattening so I had only rotis.'

'But 1 roti is equal to half a cup of rice, as far as calories go.' I am still amazed at the kind of myths propagated about what not to eat. Rice has been vilified extensively in this context.

'But I have been eating 3 rotis for lunch,' she said. 'Do you mean I can have 1½ cups of rice instead?'

'Since your total requirement from the bread/cereal group is 5 servings per day, if you were eating 3 rotis for lunch, then you should have been eating only 1 serving from this group for breakfast and dinner. Was that what you were doing?'

'Oh my God, NO. I only stopped eating rice. I have about 1½ to 2 cups of upma for breakfast and maybe a cup or two of pasta or something like that for dinner.'

'That amounts to about 8-9 servings of the bread/cereal group, Maya. Eliminating rice alone has not really helped you, has it?'

'But your cups are so small!' she wailed.

'They are not MY cups. They are the internationally recommended cup measures. If you include the other food groups, like enough vegetables, fruit, yogurt and, most importantly, the protein, you will be satisfied.'

I was used to this reaction about the cups in question. There is always a look of pure horror when I show them to clients!

'And anyway, Maya,' I continued, 'I thought you didn't eat rice, so what's the problem?'

'Well, you tell me first I could eat rice, then you tell me I can only eat a tiny amount, that's just mean!' Going from NO RICE to SOME RICE was somehow upsetting, it appears!

We worked some more on her diet plan. It finally sunk in that the rice was not ALL that she was eating, and she had to eat only unrefined rice, red or brown, there were so many other options for each meal that she could not possibly starve.

WATER

A discussion on diet is never complete without a mention of the importance of water. Water is the most important nutrient involved in almost every vital process in the body. It is required for digestion, circulation, removing waste products, building and repair of cells, and the transportation of other nutrients in the body.

One needs at least 8 glasses of water a day, more in hotter weather and if one is exercising. You can sip water throughout your exercise routine. Always remember to carry water with you to your gym or if you are out on an exceptionally long walk or run. You could very easily get dehydrated if you don't hydrate well, before and during a workout, especially outdoors.

Recently, First Lady of the United States Michelle Obama unveiled the **MyPlate** as an alternative to the MyPyramid food guide for Americans. According to the guide, at each meal:

- 50 per cent of your plate needs to be filled with fruits and vegetables.
- The remaining is filled with lean protein, low fat dairy and whole grains.

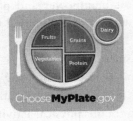

The following foods are important for women. Include these in your diet about 3 times a week:

- Soy
- Flaxseed oil and powder
- Spirulina: a vegetarian source of protein
- Eggs
- Fish: containing omega-3 fatty acids which are essential for brain function and also anti-inflammatory.
- Walnuts
- Dark chocolate: contains powerful antioxidant properties, has natural stimulants like caffeine, and stimulates the

production of endorphins. Consume ½ to 1 ounce or 14–28 gm per day. More is not better.

- Avocado: high in mono-saturated fat. Consume ¼ to ½ an avocado per day.
- Pomegranate: contains antioxidants that protect the brain from free radicals.
- Green tea
- Bean sprouts
- Wheat germ, sunflower seeds: rich in vitamin E
- Berries—blueberries, blackberries—protect the brain from oxidative stress and age-related conditions like dementia and Alzheimer's; improve learning capacity.
- Coloured veggies and citrus fruits
- Freshly brewed tea, 2–3 cups per day. Has moderate caffeine to boost brainpower and plenty of antioxidants like catechins, which promote blood flow.
- Beans, lentils and black beans—½ cup per day—help stabilize blood sugar.
- A calcium supplement daily after the age of 30
- For women with heavy bleeding, athletes, or those who participate in strenuous physical activities, it is important to check haemoglobin levels and substitute an iron supplement if required.

Questions & DIY

Make a list of 1 serving of your favourite foods from each food group:

Bread/cereal
1-
2-
3-
4-

Fruit
1-
2-
3-
4-

Vegetables
1-
2-
3-
4-

Protein
1-
2-
3-
4-

Milk group
1-
2-
3-
4-

Plan your own diet with all the food groups:
Breakfast:

Snack:

Lunch:

Snack:

Dinner:

Make a list of your favourite snacks and find out which food group
they belong to and how many calories they contain.

Don't dig your grave with your own knife and fork.
                                                    —English proverb

CHAPTER 10

REST AND RECOVERY
A CRITICAL ASPECT OF FITNESS

Rest and recovery is as important to realizing optimum health as nutrition and the 4 pillars of fitness. Neglect this aspect and it is as good as self-sabotage.

> *Sleep is the best meditation.*
> —*The 14th Dalai Lama*

Sleep is the most important restorer of energy. A minimum of 7 hours of sleep is necessary for one to be completely productive the following day. Of course, there are some, including myself at times, who survive on 4–5 hours of sleep and I honestly have no explanation for how one functions at these times. Perhaps we have trained our bodies to function on less sleep. **Unless you have a good night's sleep, you are never really awake.** Aside from feeling fatigued and petulant, your fitness and weight loss efforts suffer from lack of sleep.

Muscle recovery following strength training occurs during sleep and not during the actual execution of the exercise itself. If one works the leg muscles, the recovery from challenge and growth of these muscles occurs while you rest. Your next session of weight training for the leg muscles should ideally be after 48 hours. Training the muscle earlier will only stress it further and it will not reach its optimum potential in strength, size or tone.

Trying to train a sleep-deprived body repeatedly often leads to your body breaking down. It becomes more susceptible to illnesses like the common cold and flu. Your fitness levels drop instead of improving. You feel tired all the time, even wake up tired. Your muscles remain sore.

Weight gain is one of the repercussions of constant sleep deprivation. In an extensive study of women called the Nurses' Health Study begun in 1976, the researchers followed a group of women over a period of 16 years and found that, among other things, women sleeping 5 hours or less tended to gain more weight than those who managed to sleep more.

Why Sleep Deprivation Can Lead to Weight Gain

- One of the hypotheses is that anyone sleep-deprived is also very tired and tends not to work out or even be physically active.
- Another theory is that when the body does not get enough sleep, it may lower the basal metabolic rate trying to conserve energy, and as a result lay on kilos.
- Sleep deprivation can also cause the stress hormone cortisol to increase, in turn causing weight gain.
- Often the body cannot differentiate between fatigue and hunger. A sleep-deprived individual often eats indiscriminately to soothe an inner sense of discomfort. All she probably requires is a couple of hours of sleep.

I can most definitely identify with the confusion of sleep deprivation with hunger. There have been nights when I would come home exhausted after attending to surgery or women in labour, and head straight for the fridge. I was hungry, wasn't I? At least that was what my body told me. Anyone who works nights, sleeps less or even has a stressful life may have experienced similar cravings. The body needs to appease itself, and food emerges a clear winner. It doesn't have to be. **Once you recognize this confusion, even a cup of herbal tea helps soothe and satisfy without adding weight.**

Women who work night shifts like nurses, doctors or call-centre employees, need to be aware of the turmoil the body faces when it is sleep-deprived and fatigued. Stress is a by-product of sleep deprivation. Stress by itself can cause weight gain.

So the question arises, do I get up half an hour earlier to exercise or do I sleep in to combat fatigue? This is a difficult one to answer. It depends on what is going on in your life at that point of time and what exactly your fitness goals are. If you are genuinely busy, sleep-deprived and exhausted, it may be more beneficial for you to catch some sleep and try to get in that workout the following day or at a later time, possibly pre-lunch, in the same day.

As women, we tend to have many things to do besides just work and family. Our social skills are always being challenged and sharpened and we invariably find several people interlinked with our own lives, interacting with some of whom may not be in our best interest. As a result, we often have too many things that require our attention in a day. This could result in either burn-out, or if we aren't very good at time management and prioritization we may end up not completing satisfactorily what was essential for our own well-being.

DO AWAY WITH THE TIME WASTERS

- Analyse your daily activities carefully. Perhaps you can forgo that late-night TV serial in order to get to bed at a decent hour and therefore wake up earlier to get in a workout.
- Run on the treadmill as you watch the news.
- Run away from little miss 'I-need-your-help-right-this-minute' at work.
- Eat a light snack for lunch and make it to the gym mid-afternoon.
- Stay clear of the long-drawn-out gossip session with colleagues or friends. Use that time to exercise instead.
- Escape the building committee meeting once in a while when you know the same topics will be discussed to no avail.
- If nothing else works, you may need to forgo that extra half hour of sleep at least a few times a week to fit in a workout, particularly if you are overweight, unfit, and your health is at stake.

As you lose weight and gain perspective, you will find that your time allotted for fitness becomes non-negotiable. You work around your routine and manage to fit in something at least 4 times a week.

When trying to schedule a workout with people who already have their plates full, I am always amazed at how they are able to prioritize their time effectively. The more successful, busy and efficient they are, the better they are at time management and vice versa. The women who have the least to do in their day always seem to find an excuse to skip a workout. Their fitness hour is always flexible. Everything else takes precedence.

LEARNING TO SAY NO

When helping women to set goals and prioritize their fitness needs, what becomes apparent is the inability of some women to just say no to obligations or requests that may be completely unnecessary. Many women find it hard to refuse. This leaves them frustrated, not to mention incapable of planning what is actually important for them, in this case, some time for a fitness routine.

> Sometimes you have to learn to say 'NO, I can't do this right now, I have to work out.'

It may seem selfish initially, especially to others involved. Once everyone realizes that your workout encourages you to stay in a better mood, they may even encourage you to exercise regularly.

A number of women have told me that spouses, children, parents and friends have recognized their requirement for exercise on a very practical level—not picking fights with the husband, not finding fault with the kids, not yelling at the maid, and so on!

The 'I'M OK, YOU'RE OK' Principle

At 36, Sonia is single, career-oriented and successful. She runs her own catering business and is extremely passionate about food. She is also one of those people who understands food. Although she doesn't necessarily cook healthy food, because her orders are dependent on client preferences, she is careful with what she eats. She is very clever with manipulating the recipe to create a delicious dish with less calories. She is also very active, on her feet all day and sometimes late into the night, prepping for the next day.

Despite her busy schedule, careful eating and productive...

...lifestyle, she is overweight, plagued with back pain, often depressed and overwhelmed. Her weight is partly a result of stress, lack of exercise and, I suspect, some amount of mindless eating which she is probably unaware of.

She has no time to exercise. There is always something more important to do. She is overbooked and overworked. Friends and relatives cater from her constantly. Orders are sometimes last-minute, putting a lot of pressure on her resources. She has no idea how to refuse an order even when she knows it's killing her to make ends meet.

She is a prototypical 'people pleaser'. At the expense of her own health and well-being, she exposes herself constantly to needless stress.

'You will have to cut back on your work, Sonia,' I explain. 'You are now 85 kg, with 40 per cent fat. At this rate you will progress to being morbidly obese.'

'I can't upset people by refusing their orders,' she retorts. 'What will they think?'

'I am sure they don't think very much about your health or wellness,' I couldn't resist being blunt, 'you have to learn to prioritize if you are serious about getting into shape and better health.'

She slowly learnt to say no. She set aside time for her own workout and over a period of 4 months tried to make that time non-negotiable. She made rules for her orders, that they be placed well in advance, that she would only take on so much.

This was a difficult learning curve for Sonia. She was so accustomed to being at other people's disposal that it was hard for her to actually refuse favours. Ever so often, she would take on more than she could handle.

Her food journal entries were a revelation to her. She ate incessantly if she was stressed. And then conveniently 'forgot' about it! We laughed over her entries. Nevertheless, she realized the seriousness of the situation when her blood reports showed high levels of cholesterol and blood sugar.

Today she is careful with her food. She walks 4 times a week and weight-trains twice.

Her greatest problem was not an aversion to exercise, or even excuses to escape working out. Her problem was that she did not respect herself enough to put her health first. She is still learning to do that.

The better you are and feel, the more likely it is that you will make the people around you happy! On the other hand, when you are overweight, tired, irritable, suffering from low back pain, swelling of the feet, and are breathless just climbing a flight of stairs, you can hardly make the people around you happy or comfortable.

Sometimes we tend to accept situations however awkward or annoying they are. Weight and lack of fitness is one of those things. If you have become accustomed to feeling uncomfortable, it is almost like a way of life for you. Feeling better may not even occur to you. Regardless, it is important to understand that only 'you' are responsible for 'you'. When you start working out and recognize that it can improve your daily quality of life and functionality, you tend to look at your workout not just as a means of getting slim, but as a way of staying healthy and comfortable, without pain or distress.

CHAPTER 11

THE RIGHT MENTAL ATTITUDE

ATTITUDE IS EVERYTHING

Without a change in attitude, no amount of changing your menu or make-up will provide long-lasting, positive results. **Fitness is primarily a mind thing.** Without the right mental attitude, your results are rarely sustainable.

Nikita was the life of the party. In this case, the life of the group class. She was charming, witty and sharply intelligent. She teased others, made them feel comfortable, encouraged them, and was perhaps one of the most popular students in the class.

There was only one problem. Although Nikita came regularly to class and was amazingly dedicated to her workout, we saw very little change in her weight and measurements for the first 6 months. It was baffling. She understood diet, food groups and serving sizes perfectly. She attended all the workshops and did phenomenally well at the questionnaires. So, what was the problem?

Fitness is inclusive of a balanced diet. Unless you get your 'diet act' together, you will always battle weight and a higher fat percentage. Learning the food pyramid and your required serving sizes is not hard once you understand them. You will also feel more in control of your body when you know how to nourish it.

Nikita was in denial. She could not quite sustain a healthy diet, but refused to admit it, even to herself! She never filled her food journal. She literally, conveniently 'forgot' what she had eaten.

She worked out religiously for 6 months but lost only about 5 kg. Her fitness levels soared, however.

After 6 months of this escapist caper, the penny finally dropped. She began admitting to herself that her diet was appalling. She began talking about how she binged, and essentially expected the exercise alone to take care of her weight woes. She realized that her diet was crucial if she wanted to see results in her size/weight. She realized that with the effort she was investing into her workout, she should be seeing far better results, and she would only do so if she made the necessary changes in her diet.

This was just the beginning of her remarkable progress. In the next 3 months, she lost 12 kg, built muscle, improved her stamina and got stronger. She looked amazing.

I believe she was not ready to go all the way with her lifestyle changes initially. When she was finally ready, she was able to admit to herself that SHE was responsible for her success or lack of it and that she could achieve unparalleled results if she took that last step to monitor her diet. Today she looks fabulous. She is an inspiration to other clients and students.

STRATEGIES FOR THE RIGHT MENTAL ATTITUDE

Make your fitness routine NON-NEGOTIABLE: It has to be a lifestyle, not something you struggle with for an hour every day. If your fitness routine is non-negotiable, you will find a way to fit it in. I remember doing push-ups, squats and lunges with a close childhood friend in a hotel room in Spain to get in a quick strength workout. It becomes so much a part of your life (like brushing your teeth), that you simply cannot do without it.

Be honest: It may be the toughest thing you ever do, but admitting your own contribution to your lack of fitness or your

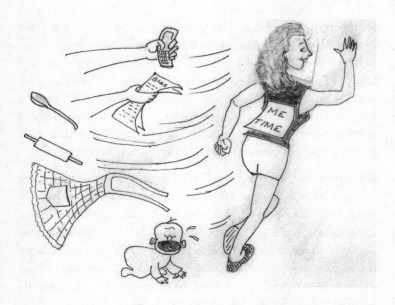

obesity is the first step to change. 'But I don't eat anything!' is the excuse I am constantly barraged with. Here is where writing your **food and exercise journal** every day at least for the first 6 months of starting your fitness programme will help you understand where you are lacking. Be honest about your food intake. Do not overestimate your exercise. That is self-sabotage.

I know women who are constantly sustaining injury and pain while working out. It is sometimes hard for a trainer to ascertain if the injury is critical enough to curtail working out, or if all she needs is a stretch and strengthening routine. This requires some amount of 'body awareness' and complete honesty on the part of the client.

Ask yourself difficult questions: Do you really not have the time for exercise? Is it absolutely essential you attend that social event, or will it survive without you? Must you have that second helping of dessert? Do you actually need to wait around to serve your husband his lunch, couldn't you leave it on the table and get to your aerobic class? Can your children not spare you for an hour? Are you still recovering from your injury, or have you healed enough to start your training? Is there perhaps anything else going on in your life that is obstructing your journey towards fitness. Is anyone preventing your progress?

Be open to learning and criticism: We are often stuck because of our dogmas and beliefs, like the idea that weight training is not necessary for women, or that it will make you masculine. Even more often we choose to believe what suits us, for instance we tell ourselves that working out at a higher intensity is not good for us simply because we are not able to work out at a higher intensity. Instead, we should gradually increase the intensity and aim to get better.

Be willing to get out of your comfort zone: Most people stay within their comfort zone. Be it food habits, exercise or routine. We hesitate to change the menu we have been used to for years even if it is half killing us. We walk the same route at the same intensity every single day, not challenging ourselves. We hesitate to attend a class for fear of making fools of ourselves! We fear learning a new art form like karate or tae-bo because 'What if we are unable to do it?' We have already sealed our fate.

Never look for quick-fix remedies and miracle cures: This, I believe, is one of the most common problems. In today's fast-paced world where everything has already happened yesterday, we want results that appear miraculously without any effort on our part. Take a pill and burn fat, take another one and build muscle, go on a diet for 5 days and lose 10 kg—it is endless, these promises of sensational outcomes in impossibly short periods of time.

Quit the pity party and start taking responsibility for your own actions: Taking responsibility for oneself and facing the consequences of one's actions, is the cornerstone of success. I see so many women who complain about their lives, their inability to exercise because of endless perceived problems. They never get anywhere because, essentially, they do not even try.

Understand that being fit is not just about weight: It is critical to understand this aspect for long-term fitness. You may start by wanting to lose fat. Along your journey, try to see beyond this myopic ambition. The chances of you persisting with it are better. Learn about and include the 4 pillars of fitness into your routine. Acknowledge that nutrition and rest are also significant aspects of staying fit and healthy.

Be prepared for change: When you make a change in your life, in this case start an exercise programme, you are bound to face a reaction from those around you. Your friends and family may take a while to comprehend or empathize with this need for change. Those who care about your health, however, will be supportive. Those who see it as a threat (for whatever inane reason) will respond to your change with resistance, complaining and needless innuendoes. I have had clients tell me that members of their family or friends complain that they are selfish and do not make time for them any more. Guilt sometimes may take precedence and you may be sidetracked into an unhealthy lifestyle simply because the alternative does not suit the people around you.

If you prepare yourself for the inevitable resistance from

those around you, you are in a better position to withstand opposition, if required. Eventually, things will settle down when people realize you are serious about the change you have attempted, and see the benefits you are reaping.

Surround yourself with people who encourage and support your fitness goals: This will keep the motivation levels high and prevent you from getting discouraged along the way.

ATTITUDES THAT DON'T WORK

- Being eternally on one diet after another.
- Constantly searching for that miracle exercise-form that will solve all your problems.
- Shifting from one exercise form to another, not because you are experimenting, but because you believe, the grass is greener on the other side.
- Criticizing science and research and believing that you know it all.
- Using every excuse in the book to justify the way you live, the way you indulge in overeating or exercising incorrectly.
- Stating, 'I go for a walk and I am fit,' and refusing to take a more holistic approach to fitness.
- Insisting on passing uncomplimentary comments like, 'You exercise so much and yet you are not really all that slim,' or 'Yes, you have lost weight, but you know, you looked better plump, now you look gaunt!'

Some women may go through several years struggling with their own weight and health, making excuses for themselves, always justifying their actions. Others may be genetically slim, but not necessarily fit, and therefore willing to make judgement calls on other women and their choice of exercise.

CHAPTER 12

OVERTRAINING

ARE YOU DOING TOO MUCH?

At the other end of the spectrum, we have women trying to do too much. It's all very well to want to look fabulous at 40, or have a 61-cm waistline. Is that feasible for you, and if so what are the means you are using to get there? These are questions you need to ask yourself.

There *is* a condition called overtraining. There are signs to identify overtraining:

- Check your resting pulse rate for a couple of days and if you find it slowly creeping up, you could be overtraining.
- Are you tired a lot, do you wake up feeling tired?
- Do you have trouble sleeping?
- Have you lost a lot of weight in a very short time?
- Have you been prone to infections, cough and cold recently?
- Have you found that despite increasing your workout intensity or the amount of weight you lift, you haven't gained muscle or strength?
- Do your muscles feel sore all the time?

- Are you just not feeling well?
- Have you lost your appetite?
- Do you feel unmotivated or unenthusiastic?
- Are you depressed?
- Have your periods reduced or stopped altogether?
- Is there blood in your urine or is it coloured (indicating dehydration)?

Extreme forms of overtraining can lead to the **female athlete triad**. This is a condition where the woman's body fat percentage drops to an abysmal low, her periods stop, her bones become fragile and prone to breakage as a result of nutritional deficiencies. Women who exercise too much, especially elite athletes, appear to be in danger of developing this syndrome.

Rhabdomyolysis is a condition where muscle breakdown leads to blood in the urine. It can be seen in people who train excessively and stress their muscles, leading to unwarranted muscular injury with the corresponding metabolic by-products being passed into the kidneys and the urine. This could potentially lead to kidney failure and is fatal if severe and untreated.

Pay attention to the signs and signals your body is sending you. More is not always better. Stressing your body will not always bring you the results you seek. Yes, you can do Pilates, kick-boxing or TRX training, but is that what your body really requires at this point? You come across this new and interesting fitness form called jukari, so you try to fit that in between your running, swimming, Zumba and yoga. Does your body benefit? Most likely not, considering the number of things you are already forcing it to do.

The duration of your training is also important. Training in the gym for hours and hours will not necessarily help you achieve that fabulous body. You may end up looking tired, haggard and lacking in energy for the rest of the day.

Pay attention to the rest of your life. If you are going through a **stressful period at work or personally**, the workout you have been accustomed to may turn out to be too much for your body to handle. I had a client who was so obsessed with her workout routine that she would, despite just landing in New York City, head to the hotel gym to get in a workout before a meeting or deadline. She travelled incessantly. **Travel is often a stressor.** Change in time zones, weather, environment, food and jet lag can put added pressure on an already stressful life. Back in India, she continued to run paying no heed to her body. She was in the middle of a **personal crisis** and this was her way of trying to cope. Eventually, her body gave in and she encountered a bad back, which had her laid up for weeks.

Body dysmorphic disorder or BDD is a condition where an individual is obsessed with a minor, real or perceived defect of the physical body. She believes she is either too fat, too thin, not muscular enough, skin not good enough, nose not long enough, etc. Very often, such women train obsessively to a delusional end and may also suffer eating disorders. This can lead to injury and overtraining. Although this is a psychiatric condition, these individuals often seek the help of a cosmetic surgeon or dermatologist in the hope of enhancing their appearance.

Most women who suffer from the above conditions are often not in a position to help themselves. It is important that those close to them take action if they suspect something is amiss.

Take care of your body, it's the only place you have to live.
—*Jim Rohn*

The body needs to rest, recover and be well-nourished as much as it needs to be trained or exercised. Balance is the key. Sometimes it requires a shocking turn of events, like a severe injury or the body shutting down, for someone to realize that they are in the process of abusing themselves. Even too much of a good thing like exercise can be bad for you.

CHAPTER 13

BODY COMPOSITION

WHAT ARE YOU MADE OF?

Bodies are not just about size, but also about shape, quality of content and the ability to improve performance.

—*Layak*

We often approach our fitness goals only in terms of 'looking slimmer' or 'losing weight'. It is, however, essential to understand that the optical representation of **size** alone can be deceptive in terms of the **content** of the body. **For instance, one could very well look thin or slim but have meagre muscle mass and a high fat percentage.** The result? From a visual perspective, a thin or slim body without any muscle definition, very often flabby, especially as one grows older, as fat doesn't stand up to gravity very well!

The pleasing **shape** of the human body is evident only when muscle structure is defined with a thin layer of fat encasing it. When this subcutaneous fatty layer increases, the muscle definition perceptibly disappears. The curve of the waist begins to get obliterated, on profile; the abdomen is no longer flat.

The quality of content refers to the ratio of fat to muscle in the body. This ratio has to be at an optimum for a well-sculpted appearance. **The body consists of various components** like bone, muscle, fat, and internal organs, nerves, blood vessels. From the perspective of physical fitness, the percentage of body fat and lean body mass, which is the composite collection of the non-fat tissue, is of prime importance.

The purpose of all muscle is locomotion and strength. Fat, on the other hand, has some bodily functions such as storage of energy, insulation and protection of important organs. However, there is a ceiling to the amount of fat that is required to perform these very functions. In excess, fat is completely redundant.

The quality of content also refers to the actual functionality of individual muscles. Having a lot of muscle is not sufficient. The muscle needs to be strong, flexible, and with high endurance. For instance, one may be proportionately and attractively muscular with an ideal fat percentage but have extremely tight, inflexible muscles and an imbalance in muscle distribution and strength, leading to poor posture and body alignment. This is where a fitness programme that is holistic, addressing all the aspects of fitness including cardiovascular endurance, balance, strength, flexibility, coordination and agility of the entire body, is vital. An individual's ability to **improve performance** is a direct result of having a **good quality body**.

This ability to improve performance affects the entire spectrum of daily life, from the boardroom to the bedroom, from being a multitasking supermom to the executive socialite.

The **role of fitness**, therefore, is to enable one not only to reach optimum body composition, but also improve functionality by addressing the other aspects of fitness.

Is there an ideal shape for the human body? I don't think so. Obviously, different cultures appreciate different human shapes and sizes. Genetically, depending on evolution and geographical location, the human body appears in different forms. The basic structure, the height, frame, size and weight of individual bones, and the quantity of muscle differ between genetic pools and nationalities.

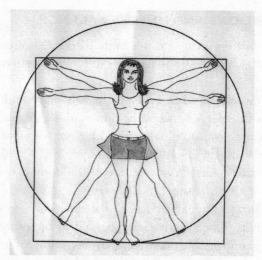

The Modern Vitruvian Woman

Leonardo da Vinci's painting *Vitruvian Man* from the Renaissance period in Europe depicts the ideal male proportions as calculated by Marcus Vitruvius, an architect of that period. The human form portrayed as the *Vitruvian Man* is beautiful, with sculpted muscles that are well balanced and proportionate. Although the drawing itself is obviously awe-inspiring and has been used the world over to represent the perfectly sculpted man by various organizations, corporates and even the medical community, I am not sure if there is one single ideal that we are supposed to aspire towards. According to Dr Adrian Ngyunen, the *Vitruvian Man* is 'the embodiment of health for man and woman.'

Much as we all may want to achieve exact proportions, this is neither possible, nor necessary. However, it helps to have well-balanced muscles not just for aesthetic reasons but to prevent injury.

PROPORTIONS AND MUSCLE BALANCE

The proportions of the various body parts are as important as the overall size of the body. In order to achieve **well-balanced muscles**:

- The muscles need to be equal in size, shape and strength on both sides of the body. Sometimes muscles on one side (often the dominant side, the right for right-handed individuals, for instance) are stronger and slightly larger. Alternately, muscles in one side of the body may be more flexible than the other.
- Opposing muscles need to be balanced in size, strength and flexibility. These are muscles that aid in opposing actions. For example, the quadriceps in the front of the thigh extend the knee joint, while the hamstrings at the back of the thigh flex or bend the knee.

For instance, training opposing muscles in the leg—the quadriceps and hamstrings—will bring balance to it in shape, size and functionality, and stability to the knee joint. Having prominent and overdeveloped quads not only looks strange, but when combined with weak, underdeveloped hamstrings, will set the stage for injury to the knee, back and the muscle itself.

The purpose of a fitness assessment prior to starting a fitness routine, therefore, is to determine which muscles need more work and training and to identify muscle imbalances. Some women may need to train very hard to strengthen their quads or hamstrings. Others may need to focus on their upper back, the lats and the trapezius, which may be overstretched and weak. This kind of disparity in muscle development could be due to the overuse of certain sets of muscles and the underuse of others, or it may even be genetic. The result of muscle imbalance is often pain and poor functionality. Specific exercises targeting these muscles to increase strength and size can reduce pain and improve both appearance and functionality.

Suffice to say, the female form comes in many shapes and sizes. Many of them may not be the 'ideal'. The objective of starting a fitness programme is to make the best of what we are born with. It is possible to improve the **shape and size** of the body with the right kind of exercises.

In order to identify the shape of the female body, one has to take measurements in 3 specific inflection points:

- **Bust**: measured across the fullest part of the woman's breasts,
- **Waist**: at the smallest circumference of the abdomen, and
- **Hips**: at the largest circumference of the hip and buttocks.

THE 4 MAIN FEMALE BODY SHAPES

Banana: The body looks almost rectangular. The waist is less than 22.5 cm smaller than the hips or bust measurement. The curve of the waist is minimal. If this body has a very low body fat percentage it would look almost boyish in appearance. Body fat when accumulated, is distributed typically in the abdomen, buttocks, chest and face.

Apple (triangle downwards): These women have broader shoulders than hips. Their legs and hips may be slim. The fat accumulation occurs on the abdomen and chest. From a health perspective, this is not a good shape to have, as fat accumulation in and around the abdomen is the dangerous kind, leading to a higher incidence of heart disease and diabetes.

Pear (triangle upward): These women have a hip measurement greater than their bust. The fat is accumulated around the hips and thighs, which are a safer place for the deposit of fat from a health perspective.

Hourglass (opposing triangles, facing inward): Hips and bust are almost equal in size with a narrow waist. Fat accumulation is typically in the bust area and the hips and buttocks. Old Hindu sculptures depict goddesses with the hourglass figure with tiny waists, a well-endowed bustline and prominent hips. I often wonder what kind of fitness routine they followed!

This is visually the most attractive body type. However, from a fitness perspective, it is more important to have a normal fat percentage and good fitness levels than just an hourglass figure. Care must be taken to avoid excess fat accumulation irrespective of the area in the body where it accumulates. Although it is true that the **pear** is a safer shape to have than the **apple**, or even the **hourglass figure** for that matter, training to keep the fat within the good or excellent range should be the final objective.

Are You an Apple or a Pear?

Take an inch tape and measure your waist at its narrowest point
and your hips at the widest point. Divide your waist measurement
by your hip measurement. You will get a decimal number.
- If the result is 0.8 or lower, you have a pear-shaped body.
- If the result is larger than 0.8, you have an apple-shaped body.

Fat accumulation will occur, irrespective of the shape of the body,
when your calorie intake exceeds the calorie expenditure.

TRAINING SCHEDULES FOR THE BODY SHAPES

Any form of cardio will burn calories, some activities more
than others. When fat is used as energy, it is taken from the
stores in the body. Unfortunately, one cannot direct the body
to use fat solely from the abdomen, the thighs or the arms.
Fat burns from all over the body, and where exactly the fat
burns is genetically programmed. When a pear-shaped woman
starts losing fat, she may become thinner in her upper body.
On persisting with her calorie-burning exercises and diet to
maintain a negative calorie balance, the fat will gradually burn
from the lower body as well. In the meantime, it is important
for her to build muscle in her upper body to balance it out.
It is also important to keep motivation levels high. Very often,
the initial weight loss may cause some concern if it is not from
the area of the body that you desire. In addition, friends and
well-wishers may comment about this weight loss and lead to
one feeling insecure and demotivated about continuing with
the fitness routine.

An apple-shaped woman, on the other hand, may start
with losing fat from her already slim legs and hips before the
fat around the abdomen and chest is addressed. This is one

of the reasons why it is important to stick with an exercise programme long enough and not get discouraged after the first few weeks.

Amla was a typical Pear. She had narrow shoulders, a small bustline and thin arms. Her hips, thighs and butt were another story. They looked like they did not belong to her. This pattern of fat accumulation appeared to be genetic. Her mother and aunt had a similar body shape.

When she started working out, she was positive and motivated despite her obviously incongruous body proportions. In the first 12 weeks of her working out, she began losing fat, but mainly from her upper body. On the scale, she had lost 8 kg. As she was training seriously with weights, her upper body began to look lean and more toned. Her hips, however, changed very little. Although there was a loss of inches, it was not quite as noticeable as her upper body.

She came to me one day teary-eyed. She had been to a social event the previous evening. All her friends had informed her that she looked gaunt, ill and old. They preferred her former cherubic looks, and anyway what was the point of all this as her hips were the same? She was disheartened. I told her, this was common in the initial stages of weight loss. Her body was typically programmed to hold on to the weight on the hips, and she would eventually lose it if she persisted with the exercise. Her friends had suggested that 'dieting' alone was a better option. They knew a good 'dietician'.

But didn't she already know how to manage her food and eat healthy? In fact, she was very good at it. She had pretty much mastered how to manage her meals by balancing her food groups, and she snacked healthy. This was one of the reasons she had lost as much weight as she had, so comfortably, without feeling constant hunger. In my opinion, she also looked healthy, fresh, and not gaunt as her friends had claimed.

Her friends had suggested she needed a special diet that would burn the fat from her hips. I was intrigued. She decided much to...

...our horror that she would now stop exercising and try to get on the special diet that promised miracles.

Two months later, Amla was back to her original weight and proportions. She had indeed tried not one but two special diets, which were obviously unsustainable. She had also stopped all forms of exercise and had joined a slimming parlour, which promised to specifically address the fat on her hips with body wraps, electrical stimulation and other bizarre contraptions.

She was depressed and, I suspect, found it hard to express that she should never have stopped working out in the first place. She has started working out again. This time with more determination than ever.

A year later, Amla looks fabulous. Her motivation and perseverance are commendable.

Sometimes you do go astray, trying new or more tempting solutions that offer a quick fix. The point is to get back to being sensible and stay focused on not just losing weight but the process followed to achieve the goal, ensuring that it is safe as well as effective.

Body Shape	Cardio	Weight Training
Pear	Flat-walking or -running depending on fitness levels; dance aerobics; Zumba	Increase muscle mass in the upper body by training the upper body at least thrice a week, with higher weights and lower reps, in multiple sets. Lower body can be trained twice a week, with lower weights and higher reps, in a fewer number of sets.
Apple	Cross-training, incline-walking or running; step aerobics	Build muscle in the extremities and strengthen the core. Train the chest, back, arms and legs twice a week with high weights and lower reps. Abdominal exercises every day, training the transversus and obliques (sides of the waist) on alternate days.

Body Shape	Cardio	Weight Training
		Core exercises for the transversus abdominis (the muscle that runs around the waist like a belt) rather than just the rectus abdominis (the muscle that runs vertically from the sternum to the pubic bone below) alone. Simple exercises, like the cat stretch, T-stand, twists, side bends and Swiss ball cross crunches, will work the core and not just the outer abdominal muscles.
Banana	Power walking, incline-walking and incline-running to build muscle in the lower body; kick-boxing; bicycling	Total body routine twice a week, with higher weight and lower reps; higher number of sets to build muscle in the extremities and keep the waist small.
Hourglass	Any kind of cardio will do depending on how much fat there is to lose.	Total body routine twice a week to maintain or improve tone and strength.

Please note that any form of cardio (of your choice) will work to burn fat. If an apple-shaped woman wants to take a few step classes a week, she should certainly do so. The chances of one staying with a fitness routine are largely dependent on how much they enjoy their choice of activity. **The suggestions made above are only suggestions and are not necessarily written in stone.**

In the seventeenth and eighteenth centuries women were represented as slightly larger in size, for example in the paintings of Flemish painter Peter Paul Rubens. Those same women would be considered obese by today's standards. American actress Lillian Russell, at the turn of the twentieth century, weighed 90 kg, and was considered beautiful. Our very own movie stars have shown a remarkable reduction in the size of their waist, hips and thighs over the years, setting a precedent for women in general in this country.

Although different cultures have different norms and ideals for body size, **a narrow waist has been found to be attractive across cultures. From a health perspective, a flat stomach and narrow waist with a strong core is most definitely advantageous**. This denotes that there is minimal fat in and around the abdominal cavity. There is some evidence that there may be a genetic basis to fat accumulation. African women, for instance, may accumulate fat predominantly on their hips and buttocks. For Indians, unfortunately, it accumulates around and in the abdomen—a prescription for health problems, particularly, heart disease, diabetes and the metabolic syndrome. **Excess fat, however, is *mostly* lifestyle-related: too much calorie consumption with too little expenditure.** Increasing your muscle mass by weight training, and reducing fat percentage with higher intensity cardiovascular activity is required to maintain optimum body composition.

MEASURING YOUR FAT PERCENTAGE

While setting fitness goals, it is wise to address fat percentage as well as body weight. A more muscular, stronger body, is more capable of higher intensity work, be it exercise or regular day-to-day activity, muscle being active tissue. Excess fat, on the other hand, is dead weight and does nothing in helping an individual be active or mobile. Another outcome of having more muscle mass is a higher *basal metabolic rate*, however marginal that may be, which in turn aids in greater calorie-burn.

There are several ways of measuring fat percentage. The gold standard in the laboratory setting is **hydrostatic weighing**. This is a laborious process whereby the body is immersed in water to evaluate an accurate fat percentage. Obviously, this is not the most practical thing to do in a gym or health club.

The other accurate method of evaluating fat is using the whole body **DEXA scan**—dual-energy X-ray absorptiometry. This is used in the medical setting to evaluate the condition of your bones to identify your risk to osteoporosis. It gives you the amount of fat your body is carrying very accurately! If any of you have had a DEXA done, check your report for your body fat percentage as well.

A simpler, but not always accurate, method of evaluating fat percentage is using **bioelectrical impedance analysis** (BIA), utilized in fat percentage machines. BIA involves passing a mild electric current through the body, which is essentially painless, to measure the body's electrical resistance. Since fat has a distinct resistance to electrical current due to its specific water content, the fat percentage can be determined from overall body resistance and body weight. Most fitness facilities will have a fat percentage machine. It is usually calibrated for the athlete and non-athlete, taking into account the higher muscle mass and weight of bone for an athlete. Before stepping on a fat percentage machine—

* Don't eat or drink for about 4 hours before the assessment.
* Avoid exercise for 48 hours before the assessment.
* Avoid the use of diuretics or laxatives.

Girth measures and **skinfold thickness** (measured using body calipers) can also be used to assess fat percentage. The latter measurement takes into account the fact that almost 80 per cent of the body's fat is stored under the skin and can be pinched. It does not take into account the intra-abdominal fat which cannot be pinched and is a very real problem, especially in the Indian population. Skinfold thickness therefore is questionable in value. Over a hundred formulae are now available to evaluate fat percentage using skinfold thickness.

It might be easier for you, however, to get your fat percentage measured at a gym with a fat percentage machine or with the help of a professional using girth measures. Keep a record of your girth at various points such as your waist, hip, upper arm, neck and wrist circumference, and of your weight and fitness levels. All these values together will give you an idea if you are heading in the right direction.

IDEAL FAT PERCENTAGE FOR WOMEN DEPENDING ON AGE

Age	Excellent Fat Percentage	Good Fat Percentage	Moderate Fat Percentage	Overweight	Significantly Overweight
< 19	17	17.1-22	22.1-27	27.1-32	> 32.1
20-29	18	18.1-23	23.1-28	28.1-33	> 33.1
30-39	19	19.1-24	24.1-29	29.1-34	> 34.1
40-49	20	20.1-25	25.1-30	30.1-35	> 35.1
> 50	21	21.1-26.5	26.1-31	31.1-36	> 36.1

> Fat percentage is more important and indicative of health and fitness than mere weight in kilos alone.

Work towards maintaining your fat percentage in the 'Good' category.

UNDERSTANDING BODY FAT PERCENTAGES

Consider two spherical objects, both weighing 5 kg. One sphere is made of steel while the other is made of rubber. Although both spheres weigh the same, the steel sphere is visually smaller. A 5-kg rubber ball is larger and occupies more space. The steel sphere is analogous to a muscular body and the rubber one to a fatty body. This is how a muscular versus a fatty body would appear. One kilo of muscle looks very different on the body from one kilo of fat. Muscle makes you appear leaner, while fat just makes you look fat. Stop obsessing about how much you weigh or what your BMI is. Instead, **focus on your ratio of muscle to fat percentage and the circumference of your waist.** You will then start looking and feeling better. It will also change your mind about the long-term effectiveness of crash diets to just lose weight and the importance of weight training to increase muscle.

Use an inch tape instead of the scale. Measure your thighs, hips, waist, chest and arms. A decreasing waistline is a better indicator of fat loss than lower numbers on the scale.

ADVANTAGES OF HAVING A HIGHER MUSCLE MASS

- **Muscle burns around 13–14 calories per kg per day at rest.** Fat is metabolically inactive. A kilo of fat burns around 4–5 calories per day to maintain itself. A muscular body is, therefore, more metabolically active than a fatty one.

    Muscles form the foundation for movement. In order to be able to move right and elegantly, one needs muscles. To climb stairs, sit down, stand up, bend down, straighten up, twist, turn, do housework, walk, run, stand for long periods of time, and so on, we require muscle. A muscular body, therefore, will hold you in better stead than a fatty one, irrespective of whether you look thin or not.

Avoid the common error of yearning for a slim body. Aim instead for one with adequate muscle mass.

- **Muscles give shape to the body.** Muscles are attached to the bones by tendons. Without them, the body would be one shapeless mass of bone, fat and skin which cannot move.
- Muscles help the body maintain an **upright posture**.
- Muscles **protect the body from injury**. They surround the organs inside the abdomen, protect the joints, and naturally protect us when we fall.
- **Muscles are beautiful.**

How Do You Improve Body Composition?

This can be done by improving muscle mass and reducing fat percentage.

- **Adopt an exercise plan that incorporates cardio along with weight training.** The cardio will help burn calories using fat and glucose as sources of energy, while the weight training increases muscle mass. Everyone, particularly women, needs to train with weights. Muscle depletes as you grow older. The only way to restore and build it is by using external resistance. We don't typically make it a habit to perform hard physical labour every day in order to challenge the muscles. The only option therefore is to include weight training in your workout.
- **Weight training:** Train with weights that are appropriate for you to build muscle. The weight you use should be such that you should find it difficult to do more than 11-12 repetitions with it in one set. Do at least 3-4 sets. After the session, you should also feel that your muscles have worked out the next day. Using the same weight month after month will only lead to a plateau in your efforts at building muscle.

- **Increase the intensity of your workout and include High Intensity Interval Training to burn more fat.** Most individuals are fearful of pushing their limits while working out—perhaps of a sudden cardiac event or the sheer discomfort experienced due to breathlessness. **The fear is unwarranted if you build your intensity gradually under supervision.** Agreed, the sensation produced by a high intensity workout may not be something everyone can come to actually enjoy. However, over time the amazing after-effects are well worth the effort.
- **Eat small frequent meals instead of 3 big ones.** This keeps your metabolism elevated and prevents overeating at mealtime.
- **Include protein in every meal to balance and stabilize blood sugars.** Eating purely carb meals will cause your blood sugars to increase dramatically, consequently increasing insulin secretion and fat accumulation. Include protein with every meal either in the form of low fat poultry, fish, eggs, lentils, nuts or soy.
- **Sequence of exercise:** If you have your cardio and weight training on the same day, complete your cardio first and then move on to weights. This will allow for excess post-exercise oxygen consumption (EPOC).
- **Exercise just before your meal:** Following exercise, you are bound to be thirsty. Drinking water fills you up and encourages you to eat a smaller amount of food. You are also less hungry when your metabolism is enhanced soon after a workout.
- **Be consistent:** Being consistent with your workout pays big dividends. Just because you work out intensely today and eat less, do not expect to see change the very next day. It is the consistent negative energy balance over several days that results in fat loss.

CHAPTER 14

SKINNY YET FAT
THE SKINNY FAT PERSON

Is being slim, thin or skinny the same as being fit? Of course, it is not. A slim figure does not automatically endow fitness to the body. Fitness comes from training the body to have more stamina, strength, flexibility, agility and speed. The size of the body, just like its weight, is only one aspect of fitness, and certainly not indicative of it.

A woman may look slim, even fit into a pair of size-zero jeans, but may have a high fat percentage. Most of these women will face the admiration and envy of their peers. They are often told they really 'don't need to exercise' and may even be encouraged to 'eat more'. They are often complacent and rarely work out. After all, isn't it accepted that losing weight is the predominant reason women work out?

This myopic approach towards fitness in general and size of the body in particular is what has led to many women exercising or not exercising for the wrong reasons. Of course, there is no right reason to not exercise! Besides the fact that

every women needs to exercise, these skinny ones may need to do so even more urgently.

Many slim women
- May have bad posture
- Muscle imbalance
- Poor shape and more importantly
- Poor functionality
- Questionable fitness levels
- Flabby bodies that jiggle as they walk
- Tend to accumulate more fat as they age, especially around their abdomen.

I have encountered waiflike young things, who come to me newly married, shy with downcast eyes and completely clueless about their own bodies or their need for exercise. Three babies and many sweetmeats later, they have ballooned into unrecognizable, middle-aged women, barely in their thirties.

How did that happen? I was so slim!

They suffer from backache, depression, chronic fatigue, headaches, anxiety and many more functional ailments that are best treated with lifestyle changes.

Most of these women have an **ectomorphic** body type. They have very little muscle mass and it is usually long and lean. The muscle could be, and most usually is, covered with fat, in which case they are called **ecto-endomorphs**.

The focus of exercise for these women, then, is to build muscle and burn excess fat.

Nayantara was a beautiful young bride. An even more beautiful young mother. After two children, born in rapid succession, her health began to deteriorate. She would be fatigued easily, and found it difficult to manage her housework and family.

When she came to see me, her main complaint was fatigue.

She looked perfectly slim; everyone in her community told her she was the epitome of health and beauty; only she felt different. She was unable to get through the day without wanting to take a nap or several naps.

After having ruled out medical problems like hypothyroidism and anaemia, she was initiated into a fitness routine.

'But Doctor, everyone tells me I am so slim and I don't need to exercise' was her puzzled response. Fortunately, Nayantara is an intelligent girl, willing to accept and follow up on advice.

She went through a fitness assessment. Her fat percentage was 27 per cent, despite weighing only 55 kg.

Initially, her fitness levels were appalling. Her 1-mile walk test to assess her cardiovascular endurance took 20 minutes. She could barely lift a 1-kg dumb-bell (it took some convincing for her to accept that she would not become 'masculine' by training with weights).

She started training regularly.

Six months down the line, her energy levels improved. She has started running 2.5 miles 3 times a week. She trains with weights that would probably shock her mother-in-law! Her fat percentage has dropped to 24 per cent.

She is in a better frame of mind. Her son, who is 10 years old, never lets her miss a workout. Mummy is so much more fun after she works out!

Suggested Workout Routine

Cardio
- **If fat percentage is normal,** high intensity cardio with regular weight training will make you look more toned. Cardio can be restricted to 3-4 times a week for about 15-20 minutes, but should be of high intensity.
- **If fat percentage is high,** longer-duration cardio for a minimum 30 minutes at a sustainable intensity, 4-5 times a week.

Weight training irrespective of fat percentage should be done at least 4-6 times a week. Work
- 1-2 body parts/day
- At least 3 exercises/body part
- 4-5 sets/exercise
- 6-10 repetitions/set.

Aren't you glad we do not live in the early nineteenth century in Europe with painful corsets, elaborate hairdos and fainting spells, and exercise that amounted to a gentle walk in the park? At that time, women were portrayed as the weaker sex and quite literally were. They even went as far as surgically removing the lowermost rib to get a smaller waist!

Today we appreciate a woman who is strong, both physically and emotionally. Weight training is in fashion, a well-trained body is cool and jiggling flesh is outdated!

The objective is not to fit into a size zero, but to improve on the body one has by building muscle and burning fat. What would be the point of managing to get into a specific size if you are not able to go trekking, play with the kids, window-shop all day in a shopping mall, or take your dog for a run?

CHAPTER 15

FAT AND FIT

CAN YOU BE OVERWEIGHT BUT FIT?

Sounds like an oxymoron? Well, it is not. In a world obsessed with slimness, it is sometimes hard to convince a woman that she can be fat and fit and that being fit is more important than just being slim.

From a health perspective, fitness is more important than fatness. Sometimes we see women who are in the overweight category according to height/weight charts, but are relatively fit in terms of their stamina, strength and flexibility. They exercise 5-6 days a week. They can run a 12-minute mile, are flexible enough to face some challenging yoga poses. They lift weights regularly, are strong and energetic. So, what's the problem? They are overweight. A number of studies have found that the effects of physical activity may counterbalance the negative effects of obesity. It is important for women to understand, therefore, that they should continue with regular exercise even if they do not see significant changes in weight.

It has also been shown that long-term weight loss may be elusive for many overweight individuals. It is important for these women to focus on improving fitness rather than be preoccupied with losing weight and getting the scale to move. This is also less stressful for both the client and the trainer.

Kaya weighed 110 kg when she first came to us. She is 5 feet 1 inch tall, and had a beautiful smile that hid her pain. My first few dialogues with her always ended with her in tears as she relived a painful childhood and an even more difficult marriage. Now separated, and raising her daughter on her own, she was fighting to survive both physically and emotionally. She had tried several methods to lose weight. She had managed to lose a couple of kilos on one torturous diet after another, but regained them right back. Every such episode left her even more depressed and devastated her self-confidence.

She started working out with a promise to herself that this time she would continue to work out irrespective of her weight.

Her progress was slow, she was uncomfortable, breathless, and did not enjoy exercise at first. Over the next 6 months she lost 14 kg. Her fat percentage dropped from 44 to 32 per cent. She became stronger, more flexible, energetic, happy and positive.

From 100 kg to 86 kg was an enormous feat. She was by no stretch of the imagination slim or within normal. The improvement in her fitness levels was, however, quite astonishing. She walked comfortably at a speed of 4 mph, did a total body strength-training workout 3 times a week, started yoga twice a week, and has become an inspiration to many other women.

At this point, we are all happy about her increased fitness. She still has a long way to go as she is still considered fat. **But now she is Fat and Fit.** She finds it much easier to exercise. She has actually started enjoying what she does and what it does for her.

Her goal is to eventually drop her fat percentage to about 24-25 per cent, but she is not going to obsess about it. Now she is not tired all the time. As per our advice, she has built in small activities into her day to keep the calories burning,

- She never asks her maid to fetch her anything, she gets it herself.
- If she watches TV, she does not use the remote (on one occasion, she said, after completing a workout and feeling quite washed out, she had sat through an entire half hour of cartoons because she couldn't remember where she had put the remote and was too tired to get up to change the channel). She has cut down her TV time to about an hour a day; it used to be nothing less than 6 hours earlier.
- She walks to do her shopping.
- She plays badminton regularly with her daughter.
- She loves music and dance. When she is alone, she turns on the music and dances her heart out.
- She has stopped stocking chips, fries and sweets. These used to be staples in her house.

Some women are unable to lose weight (fat). At least the process is so slow that they tend to get disappointed and fall off the exercise wagon all too quickly. It is important for trainers and clients to focus, in these cases, on fitness levels rather than weight alone. Several factors contribute to the maintenance of an individual's energy balance, and some cannot be clearly demonstrated. Although the general equation of energy intake and expenditure still holds true, it is not a precise mathematical science.

So for instance, two people wanting to lose weight in the same fitness programme, eating the same quantity of food, may respond quite differently. However, persistence pays. Continuing to maintain a calorie deficit will eventually result in weight loss.

Diet is a major contributor to fat loss. In July 2009, *Time* magazine came out with an article (with prominent pictures on the front page) saying that exercise will not really cause you to lose weight. I got several phone calls from clients in this regard, gleefully wanting to know what that meant. Were they going to have to cut back on exercise? Did it mean they should only diet? It had opened a Pandora's box. Most people reading that article had not read between the lines. Sure, it is easier to lose weight by cutting calories rather than exercising, as frankly even very strenuous exercise does not seem to burn too many calories (much to your disgust). So, in order to create a negative calorie balance, cutting calories from food is obviously more effective and you end up losing weight.

As explained in Chapter 1, however, **fitness is really not JUST about weight.** The benefits of exercise far outweigh those of weight loss with a low-calorie diet. The combination of a balanced diet and exercise is the right solution. When you exercise long enough, and your body becomes accustomed to it to the point of enjoying it, your focus shifts from just weight to the other benefits of exercise.

CHAPTER 16

MIDDLE MANAGEMENT

ABDOMINAL FAT OR THE KILLER BELLY DISEASE

There is no such thing as spot reduction!

If you have fat accumulated around your waist and want to lose it, there are 3 simple things you need to do:
- Cardio
- Strength training
- Balanced healthy eating

There is just no way around it!

Fat accumulation around the waist simply means that your fat percentage is higher than it should be. The excess fat, then, sits on your abdomen. For a slim waist your fat percentage has to be well within the norms. As your fat percentage increases, the fat cells increase in size and depending on where they are distributed in your body, you get fat around your waist, on your hips or thighs as the case may be.

Spot-reducing specifically your abdominal fat just cannot work. You cannot make the calories burn from your abdominal fat alone!

I know women who do 500 crunches a day in the hope of obtaining that flat stomach. Five hundred! Even a 100 crunches a day is way too many. It is not the numbers that matter, but how you do them. When done properly, even 15 crunches per set (do about 4 sets) can work the muscle and you should feel it protesting after the first 12. Besides putting a lot of strain on the spine, too many crunches will not help you lose that fat around the waist. You should also be doing different exercises for the abs, not just crunches.

The **abdominal muscles** are comprised of the following:

- **Rectus abdominis** is a pair of long lean muscles that run from the bottom of your sternum and ribs to your pubic bone below. The so-called six-pack is created when this muscle is trained well, delineating the tendinous demarcations on it without being covered with a layer of fat.

  Any exercise that curls the upper body towards the pelvis (classic crunch) or the lower body towards the ribs (reverse crunch) will work this pair of muscles.

- **Obliques** are a pair of muscles on either side of the rectus. This forms the curve of the waist. Any exercise that twists the waist, directing the right shoulder towards the left hip or left shoulder towards the right hip (classic bicycling or cross-crunching exercises) works the obliques.

- **Transversus abdominis** is a band of muscles that encircles the waist much like a belt. Any exercise that draws the abdominal wall towards the spine without even necessarily raising the upper or lower body (cat stretch) will work the transversus.

Sit-ups, tuck-ups, crunches and variations of abdominal exercises target the muscles around the waist and on the abdominal wall. Despite these muscles becoming strong and tight after working them repeatedly, if the fat accumulation over the abdominal wall remains, your stomach will not be flat. The combination of strong, tight muscles and very little fat over them, gives the appearance of a flat stomach.

It's the same story with any other part of your body. I have heard so many women complain about their least favourite body parts: fat thighs, a big butt, flabby arms; each woman has her Achilles' heel. It is not possible to burn fat specifically from one area. Fat burns from all over the body and the sequence in which this happens is usually genetically determined. For instance, one woman may lose fat around her face, neck and upper body first; while another may lose fat from her legs and hips.

Performing toning exercises that address the waist and abdomen will definitely produce a firmer midriff, but to burn the fat over the muscles you need to persist with your cardio and watch your diet.

Farah was already doing enough cardio. She had to start training with weights to increase her metabolism, thereby giving her body an opportunity to burn more calories. She also needed to focus on her core muscles to look leaner and longer.

She agreed to weight-train when she heard about the extra calories that she could burn! She was started on High Intensity Interval Training (HIIT) twice a week.

After 6 weeks of HIIT and a well-balanced diet, in which she had to include plenty of vegetables, seafood, soups and fruit, she lost 3.8 cm around her waist! Doesn't sound like much? Well, it is. Her legs and upper body were leaner and more defined. She had far more energy than ever before. She was surprised that despite doing less cardio over the last 6 weeks, she seemed to have changed her body shape perceptibly. The curves were still there, just more defined and firmer.

There are many women like Farah who want to lose the 'paunch' or 'love handles'. They believe that, except for those two problem areas, they are 'perfect', which of course they are not! You have to work on the entire body. Depending on how much fat you have to lose, the time taken to get that well-defined waist will differ. If you have a high overall fat percentage, a flat stomach will take longer to achieve. Fat has to be burnt from various parts of the body depending on your genetic propensity. It is a great idea, though, to aim to lose weight around the waist. A slim waist is a clear indication of fat loss. All you need is an inch tape.

We Indians have a tendency to store abdominal fat. We may even have very thin legs and arms and not too much fat, but all the fat we have is unfortunately stored on and in the abdomen. This has been called the **killer belly disease**. Belly fat is the most dangerous because it releases inflammatory substances that predispose you to heart disease, diabetes, high cholesterol and the metabolic syndrome.

By international standards, a waist circumference of over 81 cm for women is considered 'obese' and dangerous. In the Indian scenario, the upper limit is set at 76 cm. Similarly, a BMI of 23-25 in the Indian setting is considered overweight and 25 and above, obese. This is reflective of the higher health risk even at a lower body weight that is faced by the Indian population.

Weight-train! Weight-train! Weight-train! I cannot emphasize this enough!

> I hear these smug claims of 'I never eat rice'.
> This is like throwing the baby out with the bathwater.

Rice, especially the unrefined kind, has several benefits, so do wholewheat, bajra, ragi, millet, maize and other indigenous grains that we can boast of. Our problem is not the fact that we eat all these grains as a part of our diet, but the lack of understanding of the quantities that we are allowed to and supposed to eat. We can eat rice, bread or rotis provided they fall within the **number of servings** allowed for the day. When they are enjoyed in the right quantities and proportions, they are nutritious and beneficial to health.

STRESS AND ABDOMINAL FAT

Have you been working out, dieting and still not losing any weight, or, worse still, steadily gaining in girth? Are you anxious, annoyed and frustrated with your apparently pointless weight loss efforts? You may very well be one of those people suffering from an overload of the stress hormone cortisol. In certain people cortisol overload leads to weight gain, particularly around the abdomen. A thickening waistline, therefore, may be an indicator of other things going on in your life.

I am often faced with clients who believe they are near starving themselves, working out like dogs and yet not losing any weight. Aside from the irony that most dogs rarely work, it is with some trepidation that I approach this situation. On questioning, most individuals underestimate what they eat and overestimate how much they exercise.

If, however, it is established that you are unable to lose weight despite following the necessary precautions, it may be time to evaluate the rest of your life and take into consideration your stress level as one of the causes for weight gain or failure to lose weight.

Everyone from the corporate executive, housewife or student is under stress. How one's body responds to stress may vary. Although the biochemical reaction to stress is similar for every human being, some individuals lose their appetite and weight during stressful times, while others gain steadily.

THE STRESS RESPONSE

According to Hans Selye, the pioneering thinker on emotional stress, when the human body is faced with a stressor (or what it perceives as a stressor), the sympathetic and endocrine systems of the body set in motion physiological responses that include the release of the hormones cortisol and epinephrine from the adrenal glands. Once the stressful event has passed, the body reverts to its 'normal homeostasis'. Most times, however, when the stress is ongoing or the individual has a personality type that responds to most situations like they are disasters waiting to happen, the body remains in a 'high alert' situation with the continuous outpouring of stress hormones. These situations cause certain bodily changes that include weight gain! Research findings suggest that cortisol is the offender.

In today's fast-paced society, there is hardly an opportunity for the body to revert to normal homeostasis after a stressful event. Consider deadlines at work, traffic jams, financial crises, sick children, an unpleasant mother-in-law, school admissions... the list is endless. The stage is set for a body that is constantly on an overdose of cortisol and other stress hormones.

THE FOOD CONNECTION

To make matters worse, food, as we all know, is not utilized solely to alleviate hunger. It is also seen as a form of psychological fulfilment. Periods of stress in your life—whether a bereavement, loss of job, divorce, exams or even a change of home—can be times when you reach for food as comfort, resulting in weight gain. This is called 'emotional eating' and is a common coping strategy to soothe disturbed feelings.

Weight gain and dieting can be sources of stress especially in today's world where the pressure to look slim is foisted upon most people (particularly women) by the media's depiction of super slim models. This unrealistic image can lead to a self-perpetuating cycle of stress, yo-yo dieting, failed efforts and more stress.

This is where a food journal will help immensely. In the food journal, recording emotions and feelings along with food entries will help us see a pattern if there is one. Very often, you may be aware that you overeat when you are depressed or stressed. Actually, seeing its blueprint in your journal will put things in perspective. In one study, just filling a food journal regularly helped individuals lose weight!

STRESS-RELATED WEIGHT GAIN

Besides the combination of regular exercise and a healthy diet, lifestyle changes and a holistic approach to fitness have to be observed if stress is to be effectively combatted. This would mean addressing your stress independent of your exercise. Identifying the source of your stress and finding ways of coping with it may even involve seeking therapy.

Exercise by itself is a great stress reliever. There is something about the physical act of exercise, where you exert your body physically with rhythmic, repetitive movement, that soothes the mind. It diverts the mind from a possible stressor to the job at hand, which could be something as simple as running. Trying to perform a certain exercise, being breathless from running, figuring out choreography, can all be welcome diversions for someone who is on high alert all day. This is one of the prime reasons people continue to exercise despite the discomfort it sometimes produces. This welcome diversion is like an addiction. After the workout, the release of endorphins makes you feel good. The stress, therefore, is managed quite effectively.

Conversely, exercise may serve as a source of stress for people who approach it competitively or generate their own stress by setting unrealistic goals.

> Nina was a corporate bigwig. She was a typical Type A personality—stressed out, competitive, driven. She worked out regularly, swam, ran and lifted weights.
>
> She needed something to calm her down. She disliked yoga, she said. Her routine lacked that balancing factor. I finally convinced her to join a t'ai chi class. She loved it. I think she also connected well with the teacher. The rest of her workout was taken to a different level because of this balance that t'ai chi gave her. We slowly added a breathing routine that she did every day.
>
> Sometimes we have our personality to contend with. It cannot be changed completely because that is what makes us inherently who we are. We have to then find ways of working around it.

Mind–body fitness disciplines like yoga, t'ai chi and Pilates, which are introspective and focus on the breath, can be used for stress management. They are an ideal support system to a regular cardio and pumping iron routine.

STRATEGIES

The strategic combination of exercise modalities for each individual depending on his requirements is crucial. Some may need emotional assessment and counselling, while others may require longer and slower cardio sessions interspersed with high intensity weight training and yoga. It is complete foolishness for an obese individual to rely solely on a 'stress relieving' breathing and yoga routine while paying no attention to her food or cardio in the hope of losing weight. She would also need to burn adequate calories to make a difference to her fat percentage.

Certain foods and herbs like ginseng, ashwagandha and amla are believed to be useful in combatting stress, and are called 'adaptogens'. The inclusion of these foods in one's diet may be beneficial for some individuals.

OTHER ISSUES WORTH CONSIDERING

- Is your workout too high in intensity, or too long-drawn?
- Are you providing your body with an opportunity to recover sufficiently between workouts in order to grow in strength and performance, or are you subjecting it to inappropriate, punishing, endless routines that are only serving to stress you further? Rest and nutrition are two crucial pillars of fitness. If you don't provide the body with sufficient rest and adequate nutrition but continue to work out incessantly, this could be another source of stress for you.
- Balance your workout. Add a soothing, relaxing angle to your workout routine like t'ai chi, yoga, breathing or massage.
- Keep a food journal to track your food habits and identify emotional eating.
- Identify the stressors in your life and learn to manage them better.
- Learn to say NO sometimes, so you are not overwhelmed with obligations you cannot live up to.
- Add some excitement to your exercise routine. Let it not be another extension of your work where you drive yourself unrelentingly towards your goals. You could perhaps break

the monotony of a run on the treadmill with an aerobic class, or learn salsa just for fun. Have fun! Try not to take yourself too seriously all the time!

Sometimes weight is not all that meets the eye. What lies beneath may be the cause of the unmanageable cycle of weight-stress-and more weight. One, therefore, needs to attend to the psyche of the individual, since trying to lose weight in itself can be stressful.

Alisha was most definitely suffering from depression. Her weight issues stemmed from her emotional issues. The problem was not simple. Over the years, Alisha had gone through several cycles of marginal weight loss (mostly by dubious means) and gained it back with interest. This had left her not just more depressed, but with a lower self-esteem and also with a huge armoire of excuses that she had learnt to employ to avoid exercise. She was basically in denial about her own role and responsibility in her weight loss process.

To add to the complications, Alisha's parents also seemed to have a role to play in the whole drama. They were anxious to get her married and wanted her to lose weight in a hurry. They claimed, and she believed, that she was being refused proposals on account of her weight.

The stress on the girl was agonizing. She put on a brave face but exhibited all the signs of being depressed, evasive and resentful.

Over the 6 months that she was with us, she did lose weight and inches. She looked better and definitely felt better. I had my suspicions about her food journal entries, though. Although they seemed exemplary, I could not tell for sure whether she was being completely honest about all that she put in her mouth. There seemed to be some denial issues. She had a long way to go emotionally.

Her parents, however, were convinced that she had not lost 'enough' weight in 6 months. How much is enough after years spent gaining all that weight?

Finally, they decided that gymming was not working for her.

They stopped her from continuing and I never saw her again. It was unfortunate. She would have made progress but she and her parents wanted too much too soon.

A few things jump out at you in this story:
- Taking responsibility for your actions and the situation you find yourself in is important to your recovery. Being in denial about your own role and responsibility in the process only makes you vulnerable to more damage.
- One's health and wellness, both physical and emotional, need to be put before marriage and other social obligations.
- Stress plays a major role in the ability to achieve any kind of results with the physical body.
- When trying to achieve weight loss goals, one needs the appropriate support from family and friends. The wrong kind of interference can be detrimental.

It is necessary to carefully adjust schedules, monitor stress levels and progress, and have a positive approach in order to overcome the barrier of cortisol overload leading to weight gain.

POSTURE PERFECT

Slouch and your stomach sticks out. It is important to maintain good posture to keep the waist and abdominal area looking as slim as possible. Maintain great posture. Holding yourself well is important not just for your morale, but to appear taller, slimmer and with a flatter tummy.

For better posture while standing

Align your ears over your shoulders

⇓

Shoulders over the hips

⇓

Hips over knees

Knees over ankles

Keep the fronts of the shoulders open like a shirt on a hanger,
instead of a shirt on a peg

Draw your navel to your spine and keep your weight on the balls
of your feet and your heels

Food plays a major role in weight gain because emotional
eating is a common coping strategy with some food
items aiding stress relief.

Exercise is a stress buster but can be counterproductive
in some people. The key lies in planning the right
amalgamation of routines for such susceptible
individuals.

Keys to a Flat Stomach

Food

- Foods that cause gaseous distention of the stomach like lentils,
  chickpeas and cabbage can make the abdominal area look full
  and bloated.
- Eat small frequent meals rather than 3 heavy ones. This serves
  many purposes. It keeps the metabolism elevated, prevents
  dramatic attacks of hunger and also prevents the bloating from
  an overfull stomach.
- Diet should be balanced and contain plenty of fruits and
  vegetables.
- Calories consumed should be lower than your requirement to
  burn excess fat.

- Don't skip meals, try and eat every 2-4 hours even if only a small snack of fruit and a piece of cheese.
- Fatty foods like butter, cheese or fatty meats are not the only cause of belly fat. It is the total number of calories that count at the end of the day and not just one specific kind of food.
- Calories from alcohol seem to be a direct cause of a widening waistline. The 'beer belly' is very real! Alcohol has empty calories (every gram of alcohol has the same number of calories as a gram of fat, i.e. 9 cal/gm).
- According to some studies, drinking green tea has been found to help fight belly fat. (Obviously this has to be combined with exercise. I doubt if sipping tea in bed all day will be of much help.) The catechins in the tea seem to stimulate the body to burn more calories.
- Fast foods like classic burgers and French fries can contribute to abdominal fat as these are high in calories and trans fats, and are most often overeaten due to being cheap and easily available.
- Sweetened beverages and soft drinks can add seriously to your calorie intake without you even realizing it. Very often we have a sweetened soda along with our meal. It could add a good 150 unwanted calories to our lunch (which we conveniently forget when we recall our diet!).
- Eating whole grains and a diet high in fibre has been found to keep the waist slim by maintaining satiety levels.
- Drink a lot of water—8-10 glasses a day to aid digestion.
- Avoid eating foods with too much fibre and foods that cause gaseous distension of the stomach. Too much of lentils, chickpeas and cabbage can make the abdominal areas look full and bloated.

Posture

- Maintain great posture. Holding yourself well is important not just for your own morale, but to appear taller, slimmer, and with a flatter tummy.

Exercise

- Spot exercises like sit-ups and crunches do not target the fat on the abdominal wall. The only way to lose belly fat (or any kind of fat for that matter) is enough cardio, weight training and a balanced diet.
- Perform cardio at a high intensity to burn as many calories as possible and to continue to burn calories after the workout. We need to be a little more adventurous and push our limits of endurance. Slow walks, light weights and gentle yoga alone will not suffice.
- Do HIIT a couple of times a week to increase the intensity of your workout.
- Weight-train at least 3 times a week. Super-set or circuit the weight training to keep rest between sets to the minimum and your heart rate elevated throughout the session.
- Stay active and busy during the day.
- Add some form of relaxation to reduce stress, which is one of the causes of weight gain around the waist.
- Belly fat has been linked to various health problems like type 2 diabetes, stroke, heart disease, Alzhemer's, colorectal and breast cancer, high blood pressure, metabolic syndrome and dementia.

Stress

Stress has been found to increase girth. If you lead a high stress life, learn to manage it effectively.

CHAPTER 17

SUCCESSFUL FAT LOSS STRATEGIES

BOOST YOUR METABOLISM

'My friend can eat anything and she doesn't gain weight, while I eat one extra peanut and it goes straight to my hips!' was a tearful complaint I heard from a young lady I met recently.

Sounds familiar? Unfortunately, not all of us are blessed with a high metabolism, which keeps us from gaining weight steadily over time. A speedy metabolism helps one burn more calories even while at rest. For most of us ill-fated beings, however, the basal metabolic rate or BMR slows down after the age of 40, and then it is in a tailspin thereafter.

> Your basal metabolic rate or BMR is essentially the number of calories you burn while at rest. Your BMR is primarily genetically determined.

In order to lose weight one needs to expend more energy than one consumes. The total energy expenditure (TEE) has to be consistently higher for prolonged periods of time for the results to show on the scale and the inch tape. If one's BMR is even marginally elevated, it would help tilt the scale by expending more calories.

So the question arises, if you have a slower metabolism, are you eternally cursed with excess fat? Not necessarily. It is so easy for us to blame our metabolism, our stars, our parents, our jobs, our children, the city we live in and just about everything around us for our excess weight. There is a lot we can do to keep our metabolism elevated and prevent weight gain, lose excess fat, become leaner and healthier.

Here are some simple strategies you could implement to burn extra calories. Every extra calorie burnt counts.

- **Weight-train.** Weight training is the key to elevating BMR. Building muscle with weight training will help burn more calories. Don't just play around with lightweights; train hard to build muscle. Use a weight that enables you to perform 12 reps of a given exercise with good 'form' and no more. If you can perform 12 reps too easily, and may be able to do a few more, then you need to increase the weight used. This one is not working any more.

- **Increase the intensity of your workout.** A high intensity cardio workout, or better still, a high intensity routine that combines cardio and weights will help you burn more calories and also keep the BMR elevated post workout. This is called the 'afterburn'.

  If you have been using walking as your mode of cardio all along, try a higher intensity step class. This not only adds variety by challenging different muscles, but also burns more calories during and after the workout.

  Low intensity, long-duration workouts will burn calories during the exercise session, but the post-exercise calorie burn is not significant. As you get fitter, you can manage to achieve better, faster results with a shorter-duration, high intensity workout.

- **Eat smaller meals more often.** Eating small quantities of food at frequent intervals (3-4 hours) helps to keep the metabolism elevated. Long periods of hunger send your body into a starvation mode encouraging it to store calories rather than burn them. One also tends to eat much more and indiscriminately when one is hungry over a prolonged period of time. One study found that people who snacked often tended to consume fewer calories over the course of the day. The key, of course, is to snack sensibly. Eating a packet of potato chips does not count as a snack. That is an indulgence.

- **Avoid starvation diets.** The biggest mistake people make when wanting to lose weight is going on very low-calorie diets. The body has a certain minimal energy requirement in order to survive. When you deprive it of that energy, the metabolism slows down to compensate. As a result you are, in effect, sabotaging your weight loss efforts. Not only is one depriving oneself of essential nutrients when on an extreme low-calorie diet, but one is also setting oneself up for a struggle with one's weight in the future. Crash-dieters tend to regain lost weight, and more. Repeated efforts at crash-dieting to lose weight become more and more difficult. The end result is a depressed and frustrated individual, who is unable to achieve her weight loss goals despite the agony of starvation. To add insult to injury, you seem to be gaining weight as the body tends to burn far fewer calories (it becomes more fuel efficient!) and holds on to fat.

Many people (women more often) prefer to 'diet' rather than exercise. It seems to be easier. This is an error of mammoth proportions if you look at long-term consequences. The word 'diet' should not be synonymous with 'starvation'. **A diet is essentially a sensible eating plan that one can follow most days of one's life.**

- **Eat smarter not necessarily less.** Starving yourself is not the answer. Eat every few hours, and see that every snack is packed with nutrition. For example, a small bowl of steamed chickpea salad is better than eating a candy bar.

- **Do not skip meals.** Don't go for more than 3 hours without eating a little something. Not coffee and biscuits, but a healthy snack that you carry with yourself.

- **Eat more protein.** Eating the required amount of protein is essential to keep your metabolism elevated. Consistently consuming large quantities of refined carbohydrates makes the metabolism sluggish in addition to adding calories and elevating blood sugar and insulin levels. Evaluate how much protein you need for your body weight, gender and activity level and consume lean proteins with every meal. Good sources of protein are lean meat/chicken, fish, lentils, eggs, low fat dairy products and nuts.

- **Stay active during the day.** Activities such as moving around, working, bending, lifting and so on keep the body burning calories all day. An hour of exercise is no reason to remain sedentary the rest of the day. However insignificant it may seem, just moving around during your day has significant benefits. If you have a sedentary desk job, see that you get up and walk around at least every half hour. Stretch; go for a short walk down the corridor to the water cooler. Find strategies to move.

- **Exercise smarter, not necessarily more.** Exercising for hours and hours will not necessarily solve your weight

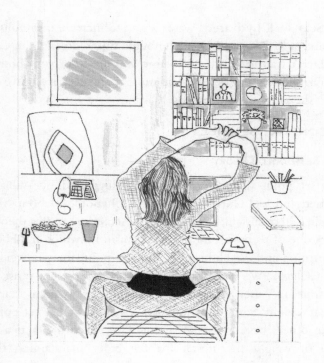

problem. Instead, it may actually result in stressing your body further. Exercise has to rejuvenate you. Aim to exercise in such a way that you continue to burn calories even after you finish the workout. Incorporate High Intensity Interval Training.

- **Make any opportunity into a physical one** so it becomes a 'lifestyle' rather than something you do besides your life. Play with the kids or your dog, carry groceries, clean, **use the stairs** at EVERY opportunity you get.
- **Walk, walk, walk.** Buy yourself a pedometer. This is a great way to increase the number of steps you walk in a day. Aim to walk 10,000 steps per day.

- **Stay well hydrated.** Water is said to increase metabolism and aid digestion. Drink enough water during the day. Don't wait to get thirsty before you reach for your bottle. Drink 8-10 glasses a day, and more if you are very active or if the weather so demands.

LOSING FAT SENSIBLY

THE SET POINT THEORY

The set point theory was originally suggested by William Bennett and Joel Gurin in 1982. It is a hypothesis about why people find it difficult to lose weight. According to this theory, every one of us has an inbuilt mechanism by which the body determines and establishes a certain set point for our weight and fat levels. We tend to hover around that weight most of the time. In other words, the body seems most comfortable at that weight. Some individuals may have a higher set point while others have a low set point. This **set point** acts as a kind of weight thermostat for the body, maintaining the weight at a particular level. It manages to keep one's weight fairly constant, bringing it back to the original after periods of weight loss. A dieter can experience constant hunger while on the diet in order that she eats more to elevate the weight to the optimum.

This may be one of the reasons dieters tend to slip back to their original weight in the long term. Dieting alone is apparently not a good way to overcome the set point. Regular exercise has been found to lower the set point, thereby enabling the individual to remain at a lower weight.

So you must be wondering, why should I even try to lose fat when my body is preventing me from doing so in the first place? The fact is, losing excess fat will help improve your health status and quality of life. So try we must, to lower the set point if there is one.

Fat loss is not easy and while losing weight in the short term is possible, maintaining the weight lost is exceedingly difficult for most people. Some of the reasons may be the body's own response to weight loss. The body does undergo certain physiological changes with loss of weight.

The question may arise, why does this thermostat not work when we gain weight? Why does the body not go back to the original weight then? This question has not been answered.

Trick Your Body and Mind

Gradually increase the intensity of cardio. If you try to do too much too soon, your body will rebel. Not only will you be uncomfortable during the workout, but you will probably not wake up smiling the next day. The aches, pains and muscle soreness may prove too much to handle if you are not well prepared for it.

Do a split cardio workout. Sometimes, it is not possible to work out at a high intensity continuously for a long time. Trick your body by performing 3 high intensity 10-minute sessions in a day.

For example

- Incline-walk briskly for 10 minutes before breakfast.
- Complete 25-30 Surya Namaskars before lunch.
- Do a step workout for 10 minutes in front of your TV before dinner.

Do a split weight-training workout. If you, for example, are doing a total body workout twice a week, you can split it up by working the upper body in the morning and lower body in the evening. This way you save time and the thought of spending 40 minutes weight-training will not seem so daunting. Twenty minutes twice a day, 2 days a week is not too much to aim for.

Participate in some form of relaxation or stretching routine to relieve stress like yoga, t'ai chi or total body stretches.

Shop Smart

What you buy for your pantry is invariably what you will end up eating. If you have smart, sensible, tasty choices of food, that's what you will eat. If you stock up on junk food (claiming it is for the kids!) you will surely find time to indulge. Firstly, the kids don't need it; secondly, why set yourself up to take a fall?

Never shop when you are hungry: You will buy way more than you need and probably not be able to exercise discretion with your choices. Have a snack before you set out. Your body is then nourished and your mind has its supply of glucose to be able to think straight.

Avoid the fried food, chips aisles in the supermarket: You really don't need to go there. Avoid the temptation to buy that new flavour of chips. If you crave potato chips on a weekend, you are better off making them at home with good quality oil that has not been reused. And no, the kids don't need it for a snack.

Learn to read labels on packaged food: It is mandatory now to label all the contents of food that is packaged. Learn to read and understand labels. Labels will denote not just calories in the food, but also the amount of fat, carbohydrate, protein, saturated fat and other additives.

Low fat is not always better. To compensate for the lack of taste, additives like salt are included in these foods. In addition, you tend to eat more if you think the food is low in fat and end up consuming the same number of calories.

SMALL STEPS GO A LONG WAY

- If you have a sedentary job, get off your butt every half hour, walk around for 5 minutes.
- Don't wait till you are starving to have your next meal.
- Understand your emotional IQ.
- Get social.
- Have a positive outlook about your weight and faith in your ability to lose it.
- Be proactive about your health.
- Get enough sleep.
- Use a smaller plate to eat!
- Stay active mentally.
- Think thin.
- Be sensible while eating out and socializing.
- Learn some simple, healthy recipes and practise them regularly.
- Salads don't have to be boring or tasteless.
- Learn the difference between hunger and thirst.
- Fill up on enough fibre.
- If you love something decadent, you can eat it. Only, eat it sometimes, not all the time.
- Drink a glass of water just before your meal.
- Associate with fitness-conscious people. The more people in your social circle are regular exercisers and fitness-conscious, the greater the chances that you will be too.

Key Points to Remember

- Fat loss is not easy and not to be taken lightly.
- There may be several enticing ways of 'quick weight loss' but question their authenticity and longevity before attempting to put your body through one of them.
- Maintaining the fat loss is even more difficult. This does not mean that an individual should not try to lose fat. It only means that **you have to do it right to get it right.**
- Cut down on oil, fried snacks; walk as much as you can; be as physical as you can during the course of the day. Eat small frequent meals throughout the day.
- There has to be an appraisal of your entire lifestyle, and not just diet or exercise only. This is because a multitude of factors feature in your weight management equation including your emotions, stress levels, personality, genetics and the environment.

CHAPTER 18

DETERMINE YOUR FITNESS PERSONALITY

A FITNESS ROUTINE JUST FOR YOU

Now, is there a fitness personality you ask! Well, it is really the aptitude for a certain kind of fitness activity. Just as not everyone has a liking for Italian food or a medical career, not everyone takes to fitness easily. This is where it becomes important to understand your fitness personality so you can improve the chances of staying with your fitness routine and even enjoying it.

Ideally, you need a qualified fitness professional and exercise strategist to guide you to make the right fitness choices for your requirements. If you don't have one, go through the following questions to understand your fitness personality and choose your activity accordingly.

- Are you a social person who enjoys groups and gatherings?
- Do you enjoy music and dance?
- Do you have an inherent sense of rhythm?
- Are you comfortable with dancing or moving to music in a...

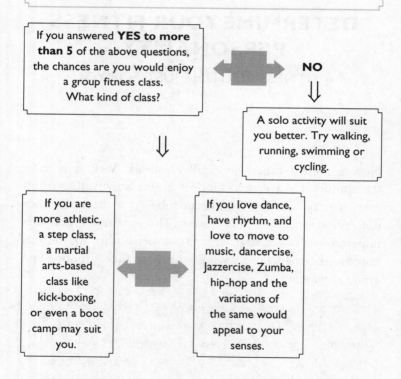

...group with an instructor correcting, watching and monitoring you in front of other people?

- Will your lifestyle and work schedule permit you to commit to a class at a specific time?
- Do you look to other people and/or the instructor for motivation?

If you answered **YES to more than 5** of the above questions, the chances are you would enjoy a group fitness class. What kind of class?

NO

A solo activity will suit you better. Try walking, running, swimming or cycling.

If you are more athletic, a step class, a martial arts-based class like kick-boxing, or even a boot camp may suit you.

If you love dance, have rhythm, and love to move to music, dancercise, Jazzercise, Zumba, hip-hop and the variations of the same would appeal to your senses.

You need to understand that most of the time the group class will not service all your fitness needs. It may be sufficient for your cardio, to get you sweating and burn calories. Ask yourself the following questions:

- Does it improve the other pillars of fitness—strength and flexibility?
- If you have posture or gait issues, does it address them?
- Does it attend to muscle imbalances you may suffer?

If it does not, you could use the class as your mainstay to take care of your cardio, and add strength training twice a week to address specific issues, like posture, poor upper body strength, poor quad strength, weak low back, etc.

Other pertinent questions to ask yourself if you join a group fitness class:

- Does the class benefit you?
- Do you feel good after a session?
- Has your stamina improved?
- Has your form of exercise improved?
- Are you getting better at what you do?
- Are you now able to manage the choreography and steps?
- Have you lost fat (if that is your goal)?
- Does your instructor motivate and challenge you?
- Does she understand your needs?

If not, stop and consider other options. A fitness professional should be able to guide you with your choices. With the number of options available today, especially in the urban setting, it may seem overwhelming to make a decision. There is no harm trying out a class if you are a seasoned exerciser. Always keep **good exercise form and correct technique** in mind.

- Do you lead a stressful life? (Who doesn't? you ask.)
- Are you competitive, driven and extremely self-motivated?
- Do you constantly need to meet deadlines, travel, make decisions?
- Do you like to compete with yourself?
- Do you dislike group activities, noise, chatter?

- Is your work time erratic where you need to have the option of being able to exercise when you can and not be dictated by a class?

If you answered YES to most of the above you may not do very well in a group class with cheery music and many people!

⇓

- Join a gym that is less noisy.
- Train outdoors if circumstances permit.
- Hire a personal trainer.
- Participate in specific stretching and breathing routines, which you can do at home, to ease your stress levels.
- Perhaps do yoga twice a week for half an hour.
- When taught by a mindful and inspiring teacher, a martial arts class focusing on the body-mind connection can be extremely beneficial in relieving stress.

- Are you uncoordinated and anxious about learning steps and choreography?
- Do you enjoy group sessions but feel you cannot cope with the workout and as a result are not seeing the necessary benefits?

Join a beginner's class that specifically caters to your needs.

You need to be instructed and corrected. Some of the steps may need to be modified to suit your needs. An experienced instructor understands her clients and guides gently but firmly. Your confidence will improve once you are familiar with the steps and choreography. You could then move on to a more advanced and more challenging class. Once again, remember to incorporate weight training and flexibility into your routine if the class does not include it already.

- Do you enjoy hard, punishing routines that truly tax your body?
- Would you prefer to combine your weight training and cardio in order to save time?
- Are you athletic and high-energy?
- Do you like the outdoors?

If you answered yes to the above questions

⇓

Try boot camp, tae-bo, martial arts or High Intensity Interval Training (HIIT).

As your fitness level, confidence and sense of adventure grow, you could try more than one type of activity. Cross-training helps challenge the body in different ways and intensities, and not only keeps you involved, but also helps you lose fat and stay motivated. The same routine every day can get to be monotonous and boring. Giving it up then becomes easy.

You need to find an activity you will miss if you happen to forgo it for a while! That is the key to a successful journey through fitness.

CHAPTER 19

FITNESS MYTHS BUSTED
COMMON QUERIES ANSWERED

The fitness industry is immersed in a whole host of myths regarding weight loss, weight gain, how and when to work out, which workout is the best for you, and so on. Most of the time these myths are propagated with no scientific validation. It seems easier, for example, to believe in a myth, rather than investigate the real reasons you are not losing weight. Here we explore a few very common fitness myths that could be preventing you from achieving your goals.

MYTH: The weight on the scale is all that matters.
A common belief arising no doubt from our preoccupation with just looking slim. Weight on the scale is not always a good indicator of your body composition or the distribution of your body fat. You may look slim, even weigh within normal, but the most important issue is to pay attention to your fat percentage. If your fat percentage is dropping with no change on the scale, it indicates that your muscle mass is increasing and that is a good thing.

Understanding how to evaluate your weight on the scale

along with your fat percentage is essential if you want a superior quality body.

MYTH: Spot reduction works.

'I want slimmer thighs,' or 'I am perfect everywhere else, I want to lose the fat only on my tummy,' are common expectations. Is that even possible? It is a common misconception that if you have excess fat stored in one particular area in your body, such as the thighs or abdomen, the best way to lose it is by spot reduction. This calls for doing hundreds of sit-ups or leg lifts to work the abs, or squats and lunges to work the legs.

You couldn't be further from the truth. Spot reduction does not help burn fat specifically in any one area of the body. Fat is used by the body for energy from all over and, often, the last place you are likely to lose it is the first place you gained it. If you have a genetic propensity to gain abdominal fat, as most Indians do, that would be the hardest area to address. Persisting with regular cardio and weight training, and watching your diet are the only means to lose fat anywhere.

Targeted exercise does succeed in toning muscles in a specific area, making it shapelier, provided that one loses the fat over that area. So, for instance, doing sit-ups may produce strong abdominal muscles, but if they are encased in a couple of layers of fat, neither will you be able to see that muscle nor will you automatically achieve a slim waist. You need to burn the fat over the muscle using **cardio and weight training**.

Also relevant are the calories consumed. You can do sit-ups and cardio till the cows come home but if you continue to consume a large number of calories, you will not burn the fat in and around the abdominal area to give you that slim and shapely waistline. You have to pay attention to your food intake.

MYTH: I will burn more fat if I exercise longer at a lower intensity.

This is a very common misconception. It arises from studies showing that when you exercise at a lower intensity, the energy is derived from fat stores. As the intensity increases, the body is unable to break down fat quickly enough to supply the energy requirement, and so shifts its metabolism to the glucose stores in the bloodstream, liver and muscles.

The most important focus in exercise and fat-weight control, however, is not the percentage of exercise energy coming from fat, but the total energy cost during that particular exercise session. In other words, the total number of calories you manage to expend determines how much fat you burn in the long term.

For instance, if you consistently burn 300 calories in a low intensity 40-minute walk, it is true that during the course of the walk the energy is derived from fat stores. If you work at a higher intensity burning 400 calories in the same 40 minutes, even though the immediate energy requirement for the workout is derived primarily from the blood glucose, the greater calorie deficit achieved from the higher intensity workout will lead to greater fat loss in the long term.

The intensity of your workout needs to be determined by your fitness levels and goals. A beginner, for instance, will find it difficult to sustain a high intensity workout. It is practical, therefore, to start at a lower intensity, for a longer duration and work your way up to burn more calories. The objective should be to ease gently into a fitness routine, not to make oneself so uncomfortable during the workout that one has trouble maintaining it.

As you improve your fitness levels, long-duration cardio sessions every day will just not cut it. If you want to burn that little roll of excess fat around your middle, you will have to push your intensity to higher levels using more advanced techniques.

MYTH: No pain, no gain.

If I don't work out hard and often, exercise is just a waste of time. This philosophy prevents a lot of people from even contemplating an exercise programme. It seems too much of an effort. However, research continues to show that some exercise is better than none. For example, regular walking or gardening for as little as an hour a day has been shown to reduce the risk of heart disease and diabetes. Three sessions of 10 minutes of cardio work just as well if you cannot fit in a continuous 30-minute routine.

This is where goal setting becomes crucial. Your goals need to be realistic and suited to your fitness levels, personality and the time available. You don't necessarily have to work out at a stressful intensity level to achieve the long-term benefits of regular exercise. Having said that, I believe you need to constantly improve your fitness levels. A good fitness programme should challenge you gradually to increase intensity.

MYTH: If I exercise intensely, I will always get the results I want.

This is not always true; genetics play an important role in how people respond to exercise. Studies have shown a wide variation in how different exercisers respond to the very same training schedule. Your weight loss and the development of endurance, speed, strength or muscle mass in response to a particular exercise programme, differ from the results achieved by other people following the very same routine, perhaps much to your disbelief! Sometimes it takes time to understand one's body, adapt and alter one's fitness routine accordingly.

Some individuals, for instance, may respond better to high intensity workouts 3-4 times a week, while others may need longer workouts 5-6 times a week. Some may respond miraculously to an addition of a regular, intense stretch routine while others may adapt well to increasing the duration of their weight-training schedule.

MYTH: If I want to lose weight, I must stay away from strength training because I will bulk up.

This is the most common excuse women find to reject weight training. Hormones and not weight training give one a masculine physique. There is enough evidence to authenticate the requirement that all women participate in regular strength training. This will increase your muscle mass, build bone strength, prevent osteoporosis and, most importantly, help you lose fat. Both cardiovascular training and strength training have been found to be vital in aiding fat loss. Building adequate, strong muscle is important not only from the weight loss perspective, but to improve the aesthetics of the body, improve posture, strengthen the back and muscles around the joints preventing backache, and improve body mechanics. Upper body strength and muscle mass in particular tend to deplete rapidly from disuse. It is important to train these muscles to keep them functioning and strong.

Start getting fitness savvy. Don't allow popular myths to discourage your goals. Be prudent, but aspire to be the best you can.

MYTH: Vegetarians cannot build muscle or perform as well as athletes who eat meat.

This is not necessarily true. In a beautiful review of research done on vegetarianism and fitness or athletic prowess, David C. Neiman examines the impact of a vegetarian diet on fitness in *The American Journal of Clinical Nutrition*. Carbohydrate and not protein is the first choice as an immediate source of energy during exercise, even weight training. When the body is depleted of glycogen, it begins to break down protein from the muscle to derive energy. Protein is necessary for the repair and growth of muscle during recovery. A vegetarian diet does not necessarily lead to protein deficiency as believed. One does not need to eat protein exclusively from animal sources to reap the benefits. What is required is a variety of vegetarian foods, including different kinds of pulses, lentils, nuts, seeds, whole grains and cereals. Although an isolated plant food source does not contain all the essential amino acids that are required and cannot be considered a complete protein, eating combinations of varied plant foods will create the necessary complete proteins. A vegetarian diet also encourages the intake of a larger quantity of fruits and vegetables, which contain antioxidants that **reduce the oxidative stress of exercise itself.**

Protein requirements for recreational weight training can be very easily met with a well-balanced vegetarian diet. Protein supplements are certainly not mandatory. Consuming adequate amounts of pulses, whole grains, nuts and seeds will fulfil the recommended amount of 0.8-1.4 gm/kg body weight of protein/day depending on your level of activity.

Your training intensity and strategy determine how much muscle you build with weight training. Consuming protein powders in the hope of building muscle, while not training adequately, does not automatically grow muscle. I know of people who religiously consume their expensive protein powders, but conveniently forgo their workout when it suits them.

The famous cyclist Adam Myerson, bodybuilders like Alexander Dargatz and Andreas Cahling, the legendary tennis players Chris Evert and Martina Navratilova, celebrated track and field athlete Edwin Moses, Greg Chappell, and the late bodybuilder and fitness expert Jack LaLanne, are all vegetarians or vegans and have magnificent bodies to show for it. In our own country, the famous wrestler Sushil Kumar, and cricketers V. V. S. Laxman, Javagal Srinath and Virender Sehwag are all vegetarian.

Vegetarianism should not be a reason for an ineffective workout or a well-trained body. Instead, to keep optimum fat percentage, and maximum strength, stamina and flexibility, the fundamental principles to follow are balanced nutrition and smart training.

MYTH: The best time to work out is in the morning.

Hard to convince someone who is not particularly a morning person of this theory. It is not necessarily true. Every individual has a different body rhythm. Not everyone can jump out of bed and run out the door in their trainers at an unearthly hour. Particularly when starting a fitness programme, try to accommodate it into the most comfortable time of the day for yourself instead of adding further stress by trying to wake up early.

Some people do very well with a midday workout while others prefer a late evening routine. A short, intense pre-lunch workout may be just right for a working person. By the end of the day, she may be too tired to fit in an hour in the gym. Alternately, others may find that working out later in the evening is de-stressing after a long day and helps them unwind and even sleep better (provided it is not too close to bedtime).

Work with your own body, not against it. More important than **when** you work out, is **how** you work out and **how you feel** after your workout and for the rest of the day. If you are going to walk around in a daze all day as a result of an early morning, this may not be the best option for you.

A study in the February 2011 edition of the *Strength and Conditioning Journal* found no meaningful difference in the amount of fat burned by participants during cardiovascular exercise in a 'fasted state'—on an empty stomach—as opposed to exercise following food consumption. What the study did find was that muscle loss as a result of exercising on an empty stomach was more likely with the body increasingly turning to protein stores for energy. Not surprisingly, exercise intensity and total calorie burn also diminished in trainers working on an empty stomach.

MYTH: I should not exercise during my period.

This is a common excuse I hear from women. This is not necessarily true. You can work out through the month. In fact, some studies have shown that moderate intensity exercise is helpful in relieving the cramps. Others show breathing, relaxation routines to be helpful.

You may need to modify your routine if you are uncomfortable. You may not be able to do your usual 5-mile run, but you may perhaps fit in 3 miles. You may not be able to complete your weight training at the intensity you are accustomed to, but you could perhaps do a basic, toning routine to keep muscles stimulated but relaxed. Stretching, relaxation and breathing are mandatory during this time. It also puts you in a better frame of mind.

MYTH: Age is a constraint to working out.

Sometimes, I hear the ridiculous excuse, 'I am too old to start working out.' What is too old? Today 40 is the new 30 and 60 is the new 40. Age should never be a constraint to starting an exercise programme, provided you have a **clearance from your physician** and are **monitored and guided by qualified professionals**.

I was recently most delighted to receive a mail from a reader who says that she is in her sixties and still participating in half marathons. We don't often see this in our country. Women, particularly, tend to get complacent after their childbearing years and settle into a sedentary lifestyle, with perhaps a walk in the park and some gentle yoga to convince themselves that they are working out.

Starting a weight-training programme as late as in the nineties has been found to be beneficial in improving strength, muscles mass and daily functionality.

The motive for exercise changes with age. **In childhood it is mostly fun.** Children love movement and are inherently active. They don't need to be told to go out and play. What is worrisome these days, however, is the ever-increasing incidence of childhood obesity. Children are not physically active, they are more concerned about completing homework, playing video games or surfing the net. In addition, the easy availability of addictive fast foods only intensifies the problem.

In the United States, the First Lady Michelle Obama has started a very aggressive initiative to get kids moving. Something in the similar vein is urgently required in India else we will have a generation of diabetics to look forward to. The **Get Up and Move Workshops** we conduct for kids at TFL are thoroughly enjoyed and looked forward to.

In the teens and twenties, people typically exercise for cosmetic reasons. The prevention of disease is far from even contemplated. One feels invincible, the only concern being, getting into those skinny jeans. Moreover, these days it is hip and fashionable to be seen gymming or carrying around a yoga mat. I meet mothers with their overweight daughters suffering from PCOD wanting to lose weight. Or young women wanting to get slim before their wedding. The question is, once the wedding is over then what? Do you stop exercising?

In your thirties, you probably start to think about losing all that weight you gained during pregnancy. If you have been unfortunate enough not to have exercised previously, then the annoying back pains, fatigue, gastritis, depression and mood swings set in, and life becomes a chore. Maybe exercise will help you. Consider it.

In their forties and fifties, women come into their own. They are more confident and able to make autonomous decisions. Societal and family pressures are not the only priority. Reality sinks in as the weight gets more obstinate and unyielding. Lifestyle diseases like hypertension and diabetes may make their appearance. At least you consider the possibility that they may. So, you begin your journey into fitness. If you are already a veteran, you will be enjoying the benefits.

Later in your life, basic day-to-day functionality is of prime concern. Most people exercise later in life only because they have probably been recommended exercise by their physicians to control blood pressure and diabetes. The incidence of falls and injury due to lack of balance increases, and the fear of invalidity and dependence can keep people active.

The point is that one does not even need to justify the reasons to start exercising at any age. It should be a non-negotiable part of your day, just like cleaning your teeth or eating. If you haven't started already, please do.

CHAPTER 20

FITNESS ON THE GO

STAYING FIT WHILE TRAVELLING

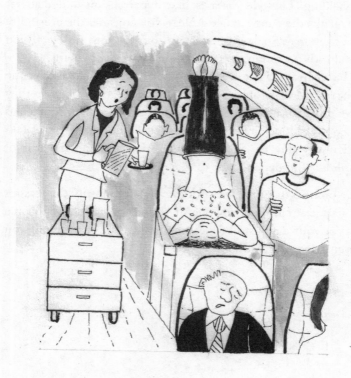

Women travel extensively today. Work, family vacations, whatever be the reason, they find themselves frequently in different parts of the world and compromise their fitness schedule as a result. Travel and vacation does not always have to go hand in hand with weight gain and poor fitness levels. Think about the effort you would need to put in to get back to near normal after your vacation. I see several women go through cycles of improved fitness and weight loss, only to put the weight back on again over a short break of indulgences.

> While on holiday, do something instead of nothing at all.

Think the 4 pillars of fitness:

Cardio: Walk while sightseeing. It is quite amazing how many miles you can cover on your feet. Metros, streets, malls, stairs—make it a point to walk everywhere. I advised a client once to wear a pedometer while she was on holiday in Europe. She clocked an astounding average of 15,000–25,000 steps a day with all the walking while sightseeing, and saved a lot of money on cabs as a result. She lost over 2 kilos that holiday despite the food and wine. Encouraged, when she got back to India, she continued to wear the pedometer to maintain an average number of 10,000 steps a day. Shockingly, she found that she normally only clocked about 3,000 steps a day here unless she made it a point to consciously walk and fit in an exercise routine.

Other alternatives would be to get in a quick run in the morning, swim laps in the hotel pool, take a class in the local gym, and so on. A friend of mine was scheduled to go teach in Paris for a month. The first thing she did was to check if she could sign up for a karate class in the vicinity to continue her fitness routine.

Her husband said to her, 'Well, at least you seem to have your priorities right! Between prepping for class, writing a paper for your next conference and trying to complete your book, I see that you simply have to get your karate class in!' Well, that's what makes her as efficient as she is.

Strength: Most of your own-body weight exercises can be done in the confines of a hotel room if you cannot access a gym. Push-ups, pull-ups, squats, lunges and ab crunches will pretty much take care of your entire body. Instead, you could do the Sun Salutation 40-50 times a day and get a great workout too.

If you are a real fitness enthusiast, carry your resistance band with you. It fits in your bag and adds no weight at all. A resistance band is sufficient for you to get in a complete total-body strength workout.

Flexibility: Stretching is easy and necessary while on holiday. Long flights, standing in queues, train journeys and walking all day can lead to many things besides back pain. Stretch whenever you can. Dynamic stretches always help to get the circulation going. I am not suggesting doing side lunges in the aisle of an aircraft, although that would certainly help you through the long haul. Simple shoulder rotations, neck stretches, forward bends to reach for your toes, and spinal twists after walking up and down the aisle a couple of times to warm you up, should suffice.

Endurance: You automatically build endurance in your leg muscles when you walk endlessly in the mall as you window shop or sightsee. Any form of long-drawn, low intensity activity will build endurance. Sign up for a long trek or a walking tour of the city—anything to keep you moving.

Deep Vein Thrombosis (DVT) or traveller's thrombosis
—the formation of blood clots in the veins of the lower limbs—
is a very real possibility if you are seated for long periods of
time, particularly if obese. Stand up and walk around if on a
flight every half an hour. Never mind that other passengers
think you have a weak bladder. **Stretch and breathe. Drink
a lot of water** to encourage you on those bathroom trips, and
certainly keep alcohol consumption to the absolute minimum.
Alcohol is dehydrating. Add that to the already dehydrating
environment on an aircraft and it is not an ideal situation.
Stretch every hour and take short naps instead of a long sleep
to avoid prolonged inactivity.

WHILE TRAVELLING, DON'T FORGET TO PACK

* Your trainers. You get some wonderful lightweight shoes
  these days, which can be squished into an impressively
  small size to fit in your suitcase. They also look great and
  are comfortable; you can wear them all day.
* A resistance band.
* A pair of shorts, tights and a T-shirt.
* Your swimwear.
* A sports bra.

The key while on holiday is to have fun while staying fit.
Your holiday will obviously be of better quality if you are in
great health with good fitness levels that allow you to enjoy
the recreational activities at holiday destinations—skiing,
swimming, cycling, walking, trekking, etc. This would also
mean staying fit the rest of the year.

CHAPTER 21

PUTTING IT ALL TOGETHER

BACK TO BASICS

And in the end, it's not the years in your life that count. It's the life in your years.

—*Abraham Lincoln*

A journey of a thousand miles must begin with a single step.

—*Lao Tzu*

You don't need a PhD in exercise physiology or human anatomy in order to exercise intelligently. Begin by learning the ropes. There are some simple scientific facts you need to keep in mind in order to make the most of your exercise. This book will make you attain your fitness goals by helping you understand the basic principles of fitness. Whether you join a gym, a class or hire a personal trainer, this book will keep you from being at the mercy of trainers, gyms and charlatans. Don't get me wrong. I am not advocating that you need to do it on your own all the way. By all means join a gym, hire a trainer or join a class, but understand what you are getting into and have some idea about the path you are supposed to walk down. Take responsibility for your own body. It is yours after all.

Begin by understanding the 4 major and 6 minor pillars of fitness.

Major Pillars	Minor Pillars
1. Cardio	5. Coordination
2. Strength	6. Balance
3. Flexibility	7. Reflexes
4. Endurance	8. Reaction time
	9. Power
	10. Speed

Focusing solely on any one single aspect is insufficient. It leads to an unbalanced fitness routine. I see bodybuilders lifting colossal weights to grow their muscle, but completely disregarding their flexibility. Then there are the Cardio Queens, who run endlessly on their cardio machines but refuse to lift even the lightest weight in the weight room, perhaps for fear of bulking up? And then there are those who only participate in hatha yoga—and that too the very gentle form of yoga where they barely break a sweat—or perform asanas that require them to support their own body weight, and are convinced they have a complete routine in place.

> If you have only an hour a day to work on your fitness, see that you get the most out of that hour. Your routine needs to be balanced with the 4 core pillars.
>
> At various stages in your life, you may need to focus on one pillar more than the other depending on your goals, but, all the 4 need to feature consistently. What this means is, even if your objective is weight loss (which should not be the sole objective anyway), you need to strength-train and improve flexibility. You need a good balanced diet in place and get adequate rest for the best results.

You may wonder how you would be able to include cardio, weight training, stretches or yoga into your routine. In your mind's eye you see yourself in your workout clothes all day, trying to fit everything in. This is not how it will be. The amount of time you need to spend on the different aspects of fitness depends on your requirements. To streamline your workout regime, make sure you pay attention to the following:

- Address your individual needs.
- Always employ watchful training.
- Keep holistic health in mind.
- Get a balanced diet plan and learn to adapt with it.
- Address other issues like stress, sleep and attitudes towards exercise and life in general.

ADDRESS YOUR INDIVIDUAL NEEDS

Every woman is different. Most of you will need cardio, weight training, flexibility, rest and nutrition. Ask yourself

- How much cardio?
- How much weight training?
- How much flexibility?
- How much sleep?
- What about my diet?
- What should my goals be?

These are the crucial questions you need to ask yourself. Each individual has to have her own set of goals and work towards them. You will need to follow different routines to suit your own objectives and lifestyle. Most often all the above questions will need to be discussed with a professional. A sample chart is given at the end of the chapter with some suggestions depending on your goals.

Usha is a beautiful woman, a classical singer and a Bharatanatyam dancer. Following her third pregnancy, she developed severe back pain that impeded her dance and practically everything else in her day. She had a slim build, with very little muscle but with a protruding tummy and an awkward stance. She had been told that she should only walk for exercise; anything else would worsen the back.

After ruling out any major pathology, we started on specific core strengthening exercises to align her spine and pelvis. The extreme forward tilt of her pelvis following her pregnancy was causing all kinds of muscular imbalances and pain. She had to strengthen not only her back and core, but also her gluteal muscles, deeper pelvic muscles and hamstrings. She also had to learn proper breathing techniques while exercising and correct her gait.

Over a period of one month, her progress was remarkable. She was dedicated and ready to learn. She was then started on a regular muscle building routine.

She loves her strong and shapely body now! She claims her dance has improved in leaps and bounds, and handling her children is so much easier!

ALWAYS EMPLOY WATCHFUL TRAINING

BEGINNER AND ADVANCED EXERCISES

Not all exercises are for everyone. There are certain exercises that are specifically designed for the beginner keeping in mind her lack of fitness or body awareness, just to steer clear of the likelihood of injury. There are other exercises that are meant to challenge an advanced exerciser who has gone past the beginner stage and is now looking at developing her body and fitness. Unfortunately sometimes, a beginner is made to do advanced exercises, which become superfluous for her: being unable to perform the move correctly, she will bring every other muscle into play just to complete the exercise thereby compromising on form and technique and courting injury.

Abdominal Exercise: Crunch vs Sit-up

For instance, the ab crunch is a simple, elegant abdominal exercise. It is meant for a beginner, but can be modified to a very advanced level just by increasing the length of the levers (raising the hands over the head, for instance) and thereby increasing the degree of difficulty.

Let us presume you skip this simple exercise and go straight for the more advanced sit-up, and that too with your feet supported, which will most definitely allow you to sit right up but only because your leg muscles are doing half the work.

Now try the sit-up without the feet tethered.

Do I hear a grunt of surprise that you are unable to do it, or are struggling with something that was clearly so easy just a minute ago?

Don't panic, the sit-up is meant to be done as an advanced exercise, **after, and only after** one has mastered the crunch with varying degrees of difficulty. Performing an advanced exercise, and that too incorrectly, does not help you advance your fitness levels or get you a waiflike waist.

When some of these pointless (and avoidable) exercises cause injury, you are set back several weeks as you heal, during which time you are unable to exercise, you gain weight and, not to mention, feel completely frustrated.

The Squat

The squat is another brilliant exercise to strengthen, tone and shape the legs and butt. Even before learning to execute a perfect squat, I am amazed at how some clients are made to squat with weights, with barbells across their shoulders, perform a jump squat and all kinds of bizarre acrobatics perhaps in the hope of seeming more result-oriented. I see the looks of agony on the faces of these unfortunate clients as they struggle with form, unable to balance their own weight, let alone that of a barbell.

> When you squat, you need to try to keep the knees from travelling in front of the toes. Sit back as you would sit on a chair. Those with longer legs will most definitely find this more difficult to achieve, given the length of the lever (the leg). Some amount of the knees travelling forward is allowed in taller individuals, provided her thigh muscles are strengthened with leg extensions and leg curls. This circumvents the strain on the knees.

Learn your basics first. **Understand the correct form of every single exercise.** Understand how to do it and make sure you know how **not** to do it. It takes time to learn correct form and the breathing technique of every exercise. Nevertheless, this is time well spent to prevent future injury and unnecessary setbacks.

Listen to your body. You don't have to do all the exercises your best friend does. Also watch out for overtraining in your enthusiasm to achieve results quickly; you may do too much too soon.

KEEP HOLISTIC HEALTH IN MIND

Getting into fitness has its own perils these days. What with the advent of fat burners, protein supplements, amino acids, and creatine, the consumer is inundated with products that are not necessarily required but promise everything from great performance to an incredible body. I do know of several individuals who have been coaxed into subscribing to these needless additions, which are not by any means cheap, with the promise of reaching their goals faster or better. Keep in mind holistic health. There has been research indicating that an overload of protein intake and fat burners has severe health hazards. In the process of trying to get fit one should not risk one's long-term health and wellness. What would be the purpose of 38-cm biceps or a 53-cm waist if your kidneys are failing?

The safety profile of fat burners has never been established. They raise the metabolic rate, can cause undue elevation of the heart rate, and may even stimulate irregular heart rhythms that could be fatal. Be wary of them even if they say herbal, which does not necessarily translate as safe. I know of several people who subscribe to fat burners without the faintest clue as to the long-term consequences of these drugs.

Ask yourself, is it worth endangering your life and health just for a few centimetres around your waist? Apparently, for some people it is! There is a place for supplements. Ascertain if you are in that place before you succumb. Do you really need a protein supplement? Is your diet deficient in protein?

Don't be easy prey to advertising, the latest fad or an overenthusiastic trainer. Nothing happens overnight, and if an ad promised immediate results you can be sure that it is clever marketing strategy to lure gullible customers. Also learn to respect your body and try not to abuse it with whatever catches your fancy.

GET A BALANCED DIET PLAN AND LEARN TO ADAPT WITH IT

- Learn the food pyramid, food groups and serving sizes.
- Understand your calorie requirements depending on your level of activity and exercise.
- Get a diet plan based on these simple principles.
- It needs to be simple, easily understandable and something you can follow on a long-term basis.
- Learn something new about food and diet every day. It

could be something as simple as learning a new salad recipe, or including more choices in your protein group.

- Learn to adapt to your own diet plan and work around your and your family's lifestyle.
- Learn the proper food substitutes. What would you serve your sister-in-law who is vegan, for instance? What would be a good high-protein snack for the children?

ADDRESS OTHER ISSUES LIKE STRESS, SLEEP AND ATTITUDES TOWARDS EXERCISE AND LIFE IN GENERAL

Stress and sleep play a critical role in weight loss and in achieving optimum fitness. If you have problems with stress levels or sleep, it is worth addressing them with a professional. As discussed earlier, having the right attitude towards fitness is vital. No doubt it is not always easy, but if seen in the right light, it can be made enjoyable. Get rid of misconceptions and myths about fitness and diet that could be hindering your progress, preventing you from achieving a fit and healthy body.

CBT—COGNITIVE BEHAVIOURAL THERAPY

This is a form of psychological intervention where the patient is taught to change her way of thinking from negative to positive. Research has found CBT to be effective when used in combination with diet and exercise to help individuals lose weight.

Much of the weight gain and failure to lose weight has to do with the workings of the mind, exemplified by stress, anger, negative thinking and depression. Psychological intervention is helpful in these cases. The client is taken through sessions of CBT to help her understand the thought process that is holding her back from success. She is then coached to change her thinking process to help achieve weight loss.

> Before you start on any kind of fitness routine: Get a health appraisal from your physician, especially if you are over 40 years of age or suffer from any medical condition.

Ask yourself this question: are you in it for the long haul, or is this yet another attempt at quick weight loss? If you answered 'long haul', then remember that it may be hard at times but it is well worth the effort.

You may need to do a few baseline blood tests to ascertain blood sugar, haemoglobin, cholesterol and thyroid profile, and have your blood pressure and vitals checked. You may also need to undergo a stress test.

Choose Your Gym Carefully

Most commonly, one tends to choose a gym facility that is close to either work or home for convenience. That makes sense as one need waste as little time as possible on travel.

Above all, your gym needs to be hygienic and well lit.

The trainers need to be of a good calibre, certified and supervised by a qualified individual.

Are the staff helpful and supportive?

Are they able to answer your questions sensibly and guide you through your routines?

Are they constantly trying to sell you packages that you may not necessarily require but seem to boost the economy of the facility?

The volume of music needs to be kept moderate to low.

The equipment should be of a very high quality and from a reputed company. Several very good companies make excellent...

...machines. They keep the biomechanics of the body, safety, usage and wear and tear in mind when designing equipment. Poor quality machines can cause more harm than good. A treadmill with poor shock absorption can cause injury to the knees. Weight-training machines that are poorly designed can have detrimental effects, like back strain.

The gym facility should include clean showers, changing rooms and lockers.

Facilities offering massage, steam and sauna are superfluous. They are not mandatory in a gym and certainly don't aid in weight loss.

GO THROUGH A FITNESS ASSESSMENT

A fitness assessment should include

- Height, weight, fat percentage, blood pressure and pulse.
- A recording of your girth measurements at various points.
- Tests for your cardiovascular endurance, strength and flexibility.

Fitness Parameter	Sample Tests
Cardiovascular Fitness	1-mile walk test
	1.5-mile run test
	Step test
	Swim test
Strength	1 rep max
	12 rep max for various major muscles like the shoulders, chest, back, legs, etc.
	Core strength
Flexibility	Sit-and-reach test
	Shoulder rotation test
Body Composition	Girth circumferences
	Body fat percentage
	Weight on scale
	BMI
	Waist hip ratio

The fitness assessment is not designed to be judgemental, or worse, to ridicule your current size or health status. It is only a baseline evaluation from which you can work towards improving your health status and fitness. If one does not assess and establish the baseline values, how is one to identify progress?

In your initial fitness assessment, let's assume you score 19 minutes for your 1-mile walk test. That is an incredibly long time. After a month of training, if your reassessment on the 1-mile walk is reduced to 14 minutes, you know you have made remarkable progress in your cardiovascular fitness, even if you have not lost much weight. This is immensely encouraging to many clients, especially those who do not see rapid weight loss and would otherwise be inclined to be discouraged.

GOAL SETTING

You will then need to go through a goal setting exercise with a qualified professional to help you understand what you need to work towards in your fitness routine.

Goals should be S.M.A.R.T.

S—Specific—Be very specific about what you intend to try to achieve—'I want to lose 2 kg in 3 weeks,' as opposed to 'I want to lose weight.'

M—Measurable—Your goals should be such that they can be easily and subjectively measured. 'I want to become slim,' is not a measurable goal. You need to use values like your waist measure or fat percentage, which you can use as a definitive measure to assess your results. A goal like, 'I want to lose 2 cm around my waist,' is a measurable goal. 'I want to become slim around my waist,' is not.

A—Attainable—Although almost anything is possible if you set your mind to it, set goals that are attainable. Idealistic goals only lead to frustration and failure to persist with your fitness routine. 'I want to lose 20 kg in the next 2 months,' may be a lofty goal, but is it practical? More importantly, is it advisable from a heath perspective?

R—Realistic—Be realistic about what you propose to do to achieve your goal. 'I will exercise 4 hours a day, 6 days a week,' is not a realistic claim. You have to consider your lifestyle, your family, your work timings, and so on, to figure out how much you can realistically do. In order to achieve your goal you have to plan your approach sensibly, prepare for setbacks and then proceed. I get women who, in their initial enthusiasm, overcommit despite being told otherwise. They then begin to realize their folly, as they are unable to keep up to the schedule or fall injured. This only serves to set them back and prevents progress.

T—Time-bound—You have to set a time frame for the goal. Being vague about time leads to an equally vague fitness routine that does not get you anywhere in particular.

Several things need to fall into place when we set out on a journey into fitness. Food management takes a while to kick in. The body rebels and sulks when you eat healthy. You may oscillate between some very good eating days and some absolutely horrible ones. You learn how to use every excuse in the book and some more to get around regular exercise and good food habits. The key is to keep going.

Get Yourself Some Training Gear

- Tracks/tights/shorts made of good quality stretchable cotton/lycra.
- T-shirts made of a similar fabric or the kind that wicks away sweat and keeps you dry. Most sports companies make them these days.
- A great quality sports bra is absolutely essential for women. See that it fits well.
- Well-supported shoes, preferably cross-trainers or running shoes if you intend to, and more importantly are allowed to, run.

It is worth spending money on good quality training gear. It not only keeps you comfortable, but also protects from injury.

Gym Bag Essentials

- Water
- iPod
- Yoga mat
- Baby wipes to wipe sweat, or a fresh towel
- Hand sanitizer
- Extra pair of socks
- Extra T-shirt
- Extra shorts/tights
- Weight-training gloves
- Change of clothes (if you need to shower and go out/to work)
- Rubber slippers (if you need to shower in the gym)
- Moisturizer, kohl, lipstick (if you need to rush to a meeting just after a workout)
- Food and exercise journal
- 1 or 2 energy bars
- A fruit

SUGGESTIONS FOR YOUR APPROACH TO YOUR FITNESS GOALS

If you need to lose fat, the important thing is to move as much as possible. Exercise is what you do in your scheduled hour. Besides the exercise, walk as much as possible.

Women requiring to gain muscle need to focus on their diet. No amount of exercise will increase muscle mass unless they are properly nourished with adequate protein intake. Keep your protein choices simple and low in saturated fat as far as possible. These women may require a protein supplement but need to be monitored while on it. Your weight training needs to be hard and heavy, training 1 or 2 body parts every day, performing 3-4 exercises per body part and completing at least 5 sets of each exercise. The cardio cannot be neglected, but needs to be shorter and intense. This calls into play the fast twitch muscles and improves the lactate threshold. Keeping the duration shorter prevents unnecessary muscle loss. HIIT is another option at least twice a week. Stretch every day, keeping those well-worked muscles supple. Rest for a minimum of 8 hours to gain the benefits of the weight training. Anything less and you might be undoing the work you have put in so far.

Exercise can work to relieve stress if used properly. A lower intensity cardio routine is recommended. For high-stressed individuals who are Type A personalities, competitive and result-oriented, you could go into your workout with the objective of expending all that excess energy. That repetitive running motion on the treadmill or on the road, and the sheer physical energy it requires, takes your mind off a stressful day. Follow that up with a breathing, relaxation and stretching routine. Short yoga routines 2-3 times a week will help balance the stress and high-energy workouts, and aid flexibility. Train with

My Goal	Cardio	Weight Training	Flexibility	Nutrition	Rest
Fat Loss	45 minutes × 6 days a week. Moderate intensity. Borg scale 5-6.	Twice a week total body workout in the form of a circuit, or super-set exercises so that there is minimal rest between exercises, keeping heart rate elevated.	Stretch every day for about 10 minutes.	Total calorie intake approximately 15 per cent less than your actual calorie requirement.	6-8 hours
Muscle Gain	20 minutes × 4 times a week. High Intensity. Borg scale 6-8.	Every day—1 to 2 body parts/day. At least 3 exercises per body part; 5-8 sets per exercise. Do the exercises slowly and rest for about a minute between sets.	Every day 15 minutes.	Total calorie intake approximately 15 per cent more than your actually calorie requirement. Protein requirement of 30 per cent of your total calorie intake.	Minimum 7-8 hours
Stress Relief	30 Minutes × 6 days a week. Lower intensity on most days. Borg scale 5-7	Twice a week total body workout: 1-2 exercises per body part, 3 sets, 12 reps. Perform exercises slowly, rest 30-40 seconds between sets. Breathe.	Every day 20-30 minutes. Add meditation, breathing and/ or yoga.	Calorie requirement to maintain weight. Consume oily fish/ flaxseed oil and powder, green tea, plenty of fruit and whole grains.	Minimum 8 hours of deep sleep
Weight and Fitness Maintenance	5 times a week: twice a week HIIT at Borg scale 7-9; longer-duration slower workouts twice a week, including an interesting step or dance aerobic class for fun and variety on one or two days.	Twice a week whole body routine: 2 exercises per body part, 4 sets of 12 reps each.	Every day 10 minutes.	Balanced diet with required calories.	6-8 hours

These are suggestions only. You will still need professional help to identify individual requirements.

weights twice a week. The total body workout needs to be slow and focused. Sleep is essential to combat the stress. Very often, a stressful life makes deep sleep difficult. Working out every day will help you sleep better, provided the workout is not close to bedtime, at which point it can become counterproductive.

If you are already fit and well within your recommended weight and fat percentage, you need to maintain that fitness level. That takes work too. At least half an hour of cardio 5 days a week is required. Include HIIT at least twice a week to challenge yourself and push your limits. Do a slower-paced workout on the other days. Include a fun class to add variety. Weight training can be restricted to even twice a week, provided the whole body is worked out on those two days. Stretch every day.

These recommendations are obviously generalized. Every woman is different, and even within these guidelines she could have varied needs. For instance, if time is a constraint, combine your weight training with cardio in a HIIT routine.

A proper exercise strategy is key to being able to manage your fitness effectively, not just for the best results but to ensure the minimum investment of time and minimum injury.

CHAPTER 22

EXERCISE STRATEGY

WORKING OUT MINDFULLY

With the exciting options available for fitness, it is almost impossible for the laywoman to figure out how to manage her fitness schedule and what exactly to incorporate into it. Professionals from particular fields of fitness such as yoga, Pilates, bodybuilding and kick-boxing will also be biased in their preferences.

Ideally, however, you have to include what you require specifically for your body and lifestyle. It may be a combination of incline-walking, cycling, yoga and basic weight training. Alternatively, it may be Zumba, running, stretches and weight training addressing specific muscle imbalances. The whole package has to suit your individual needs.

An **exercise strategist** should be able to put this together for you. There are several factors that feature in planning a routine for an individual:

- Age
- Medical history
- Goals

- Managing time
- Physical requirements
- Safety

Age: There are certain restrictions for exercise that come with age, especially if you are new to fitness. Most often, the objective of fitness is very different for a 70-year-old woman and a 20-year-old. This needs to be kept in mind. I don't know too many 70-plus women who would walk into my room and say, I want to lose this little flab around my waist. I do know one such charming lady though, and she is extraordinary. Mostly, one is dealing with ailments and managing their day-to-day functionality at that stage. I also know of some women over the age of 60 who would put a 25-year-old to shame, but these are exceptions to the rule.

Medical history: It is important to uncover the medical history before making schedules. There are restrictions for those with high blood pressure, diabetes, a hernia (repaired or otherwise), a heart condition, extreme obesity, arthritis, varicose veins, spondylosis, thyroid problems; the list is endless. A woman's past history of surgery, pregnancy, previous history of injury, back pain, etc. are also important.

The objective of exercise is to gain health not endanger it. Flawed training schedules, the use of incorrect weights while weight-training, or prescribing an otherwise harmless exercise to someone who should avoid it for various reasons could potentially lead to problems. All this can be ascertained only after a proper history taking and counselling session with a client.

Goals: Very often a client's goal does not match her potential. She may want to lose 20 kilos, but can she realistically do so and that, too, in the proposed time? Goal setting has to be done painstakingly with the complete involvement of the client.

One needs to analyse what exactly the client is willing to **invest in terms of time and effort** to reach her goal. A strategist should be able to tell you exactly what it is going to take to get there and **if the effort is worth the risks involved.** For instance, you may be willing to starve yourself half to death and train for hours in a day, but is that going to be worth your while taking into consideration the various other aspects of your life? Can a working woman, who is the fulcrum of her family and a major source of income, afford to risk injury with an unnecessarily strenuous workout? Is that really necessary?

Time frames are important in setting goals. If what you need is long-term results that serve you well into your later years, your routine has to be designed accordingly. If you want to train for a marathon in 6 months, your routine has to be managed in view of that.

Managing time: Everyone is short of time. An exercise strategist should be able to advise you about the best possible routine in the shortest possible time in the most effective manner. At the same time, your exercise routine should address all your special needs such as, perhaps, your poor hamstring strength, incorrect posture, or the fact that you are seated all day at your desk which in itself creates a whole host of physical troubles. Essentially, the strategist needs to design workouts for **better investment of time**. You can't possibly hope to include one long hour of yoga, and another hour of cardio when you are short of time. **How can you best incorporate both and obtain the best benefits without wasting too much time?** That should be ascertained by an exercise strategist.

Physical requirements: Specific physical issues need to be taken into consideration while strategizing. For instance, if you have skinny legs you should be incline-walking not flat surface-walking in order that you do not deplete leg muscle while doing your cardio.

Correcting muscle imbalance, posture and functionality has to be part of your routine. You should be able to cover everything from your own weight loss goals to the correction of poor upper back or core strength, to relieving your stress through your routine. All this in the time available.

An exercise strategist is also like an **architect for the human body**, designing routines to best suit that one individual woman's body. Do you need to lose fat, build muscle, correct posture or functionality or improve cardiovascular fitness? Do you have a skinny upper body and a voluptuous lower? Depending on these needs, the routine has to serve its purpose. It is pointless investing hours madly running on the treadmill to lose weight when what you really need to focus on is building muscle and correcting posture. Essentially, what this means is that you are investing a phenomenal amount of time on an unnecessary activity to receive returns that you don't truly require and that don't necessarily benefit you. That seems like a **wasted investment**, does it not?

Safety: The primary concern for exercise strategy is safety. If you don't really need to perform a sit-up and potentially injure your back when you can just as well tone your abs using the Swiss ball, then you should use the ball. If you do not need to run and potentially risk injury to your knees, and can speed-walk or incline-walk instead to burn the same number of calories, then you should not be advised to run. *There is absolutely no reason why anyone should be exposed to the risk of* *injury in the hope of getting better results.* You could instead land yourself in a hospital bed with a sprained back that would cost you money and valuable time.

Planning a routine for a client is an art and a science. Her body has to be respected. Gaining an insight into her real needs, including her psychological ones, is worth the time and effort spent in an initial counselling session.

I ask women sometimes, why are you doing what you are doing, and they have no idea or say, 'My trainer told me to,' or worse still, 'My best friend is doing it, so I thought I should.'

Exercise strategy, therefore, is different from just planning a fitness routine. Any trainer can do that. A strategy has to take into account the finer nuances of your life, and design your fitness, rest and diet to best benefit every aspect of your life.

In addition to an exercise routine being designed for you, you really need to get involved with your own routine and not be dependent on trainers or others all the time. As I said, it is not difficult to learn the exercises and principles behind them if you actually attempt to do so. The human body is an example of exceptional structural design. We manage to destroy it quite purposefully with our lifestyle. Although, it is not impossible to get it back on track. What this requires is some commitment and clever exercise strategy.

CHAPTER 23

THE TEN COMMANDMENTS OF FITNESS

SIMPLE RULES TO LIVE BY

1. Thou shalt cardio-train 20–40 minutes a day, 5 days a week.
2. Thou shalt not fear weight training, but train with weights at least 2-3 times a week.
3. Thou shalt stretch every day for about 10–15 minutes.
4. Thou shalt not undertake starvation diets, use gimmicks or partake in unhealthy practices.
5. Thou shalt include all the food groups in thy diet.
6. Thou shalt not try to mimic thy best friend's or neighbour's fitness schedule or diet.
7. Thou shalt not follow the latest fitness trends without first checking their safety and efficacy.
8. Thou shalt drink at least 8-10 glasses of water a day and restrict alcohol and sweetened beverages.
9. Thou shalt have adequate rest.
10. Thou shalt breathe, smile, have fun and not take thyself too seriously all the time.

Thou art unique.

ACKNOWLEDGEMENTS

To the many wonderful people who have contributed to the making of this book, I would like to offer my sincere gratitude:

Firstly, my late father, Raghavan Nambiar, for giving me the freedom and encouragement to live life on my own terms and choose my passion, without which this book would not exist. My mother, Dr Indira Nambiar, for being the extraordinary woman she is, whose influence on me is far more than I can comprehend, and who is a living example to me of how fitness can enhance the quality of one's life. The rest of my family for always being there for me.

Layak, who encouraged me to extend my medical practice to fitness. Thank you for being a constant source of inspiration, for your unfailing presence and love.

The staff and my assistants at my hospital in Ooty who make my work as seamless as possible. Senthil Murugesan and Murugan Kasi, trainers at the TFL Fitness Studio in Chennai, for being such a great support in helping me run my fitness facility. My loyal patients for accommodating my crazy schedules and travel.

Nirmala Lakshman for her encouragement and support; David Davidar for all his help and valuable advice; Madhavi Ravindranath and Anita Deviah for painstakingly going through the preliminary drafts of the manuscript; Pradeep Reddy and Sangeeta Sundaram for their constructive feedback; and Ratika and Amitabha Bagchi for their guidance.

Swathy Mandana for her enthusiasm and personal involvement with the illustrations in the book.

Rupa Publications for believing in my maiden venture; and my beautiful editors Pradipta Sarkar and Aishwarya Iyer, for their dynamic editing of the book.

And finally, all my students and fitness clients who have inspired me to write this book. Witnessing their fitness evolve and quality of life improve has only validated my belief in the need for fitness in everyday life.

APPENDIX I

THE ASIAN RECOMMENDATION FOR BMI BY THE WHO

BMI	
< 16	Severely underweight
16.0-16.9	Moderately underweight
17.0-18.49	Mildly underweight
18.5-24.9	Normal range
> 25	Overweight
25-29.9	Preobese
>30	Obese
30-34.9	Obese class 1
35-39.9	Obese class 2
>40	Obese class 3

Source: WHO Expert Consultation, 'Appropriate Body-Mass Index for Asian Populations and Its Implications for Policy and Intervention Strategies', *The Lancet*, 363 (2004).

APPENDIX II

MEASURING INTENSITY USING THE RESTING HEART RATE

(See chapter 5)

This method for figuring intensity takes individual differences into consideration. Here is one of them:

1. Subtract age from 220 to find **maximum heart rate (MHR)**.
2. Subtract resting heart rate (see below) from maximum heart rate to determine **heart rate reserve** (HRR).
3. Take 70 per cent of heart rate reserve to determine **heart rate raise**.
4. Add heart rate raise to resting heart rate to find **target heart rate**.

For example, a **70 per cent intensity for a 30-year-old** is calculated as follows:

$220 - 30 = 190$ (MHR)

If resting heart rate (RHR) is 70 bpm, then $190 - 70 = 120$ (HRR)

70 per cent of HRR = 84 bpm heart rate raise

Target heart rate = heart rate raise + RHR = 84 + 70

=154 bpm

APPENDIX III

HOW DO YOU EVALUATE HOW MANY CALORIES YOU BURN WHILE WORKING OUT?

If you don't have the MET denoted on your cardio machine, or if you are not using a machine, how do you calculate the number of calories you are expending from physical activity? Simply multiply your body weight in kilograms by the MET value (which is noted in the chart below) and the duration of the activity (in hours: take the number of minutes you exercise and divide by 60).

For example, you weigh 60 kg and you bike at a value of 4 MET for 40 minutes, you have expended the following number of calories:

4 (MET) x 60 (kg) x (40/60) (hours) = 160 calories

MET VALUES FOR SPECIFIC ACTIVITIES

Type of Activity	Description	METs
Bicycling	10 mph—leisurely pace	4
	10-11.9 mph	6
	12-13.9 mph	8
Aerobics	Low impact, low intensity	5
	High intensity	7

Type of Activity	Description	METs
	Step 15-20 cm	8.5
	Jazzercise	6
	Ski machine	7
	Stair master	9
	Water aerobics	4
Running	Jog/walk combination (jogging combination of less than 10 min)	6
	Jogging 5 mph	9
	Jogging 6 mph	10
	Jogging 6.7 mph	11
	Jogging 7 mph	11.5
	Jogging 7.5 mph	12.5
	Jogging 8 mph	13.5
	Jogging 8.6 mph	14
	Jogging 9 mph	15
	Jogging 10 mph	16
Badminton	Social	4.5
	Competitive	7
Basketball	Social	6
	Competitive	8
Football	Competitive	9
Other games	Golf	4.5
	Golf, carrying the clubs	5.5
	Hockey	8
	Horseback riding	4
	Rugby	10
	Rock climbing, ascending rock	11
	Rope jumping—fast	12
	Rope jumping—moderate	10
	Rope jumping—slow	8

Type of Activity	Description	METs
	Soccer	10
	Squash	12
	Table tennis	4
	T'ai chi	4
	Tennis general	7
	Tennis singles	8
	Track and field (shot-put, discus, hammer throw)	4
	Track and field (high jump, long jump, javelin, pole vault)	6
	Track and field (steeplechase, hurdles)	10
	Backpacking	7
Walking	Less than 2 mph—level ground	2
	3 mph—level ground	3.3
	3.5—level ground	3.8
	4 mph—level ground	5
	4.5 mph—level ground	6.3
	3.5 mph—uphill	6
Swimming	Freestyle: fast, vigorous effort	10
	Freestyle: slow to moderate pace	7
	Backstroke	7
	Breaststroke, general	10
	Butterfly, general	11

Source: Ainsworth, B. E. et al, 'Compendium of Physical Activities: An Update of Activity Codes and MET Intensities', Medicine and Science in Sport and Exercise (2000), S499.

APPENDIX IV
PROTEIN CONTENT

PROTEIN CONTENT OF SOME COMMON FOODS

Food Item	Quantity	Protein Content
Soybeans	100 gm dry	35 gm
Kidney beans	100 gm dry	21 gm
Lentils	100 gm dry	26 gm
Pumpkin seeds	100 gm dry	32 gm
Walnuts	¼ cup	5 gm
Peanuts	100 gm dry	23 gm
Almonds	100 gm	22 gm
Flaxseeds	100 gm	19 gm
Oats	100 gm	16 gm
Cereal	1 cup	8 gm
Roast chicken	28 gm	7 gm
Roast beef	28 gm	7 gm
Fish	28 gm	7 gm
Egg	1 whole	7 gm
Egg white	1	4 gm

PROTEIN CONTENT OF FOOD CHOICES FROM THE MILK GROUP

Food Item	Quantity	Protein Content
Milk	1 cup	6.3 gm
Low fat yogurt	1 cup	8 gm
Cheese (cheddar)	28 gm	7 gm
Soy milk	200 ml	6 gm
Cottage cheese	¼ cup	7 gm
Tofu	100 gm	17 gm

PROTEIN CONTENT OF FOOD CHOICES FROM THE BREAD/CEREAL GROUP

Food Item	Quantity	Protein Content
Potato	100 gm	4 gm
Red rice	100 gm	7.5 gm
White rice	100 gm	6.5 gm
Hempseed	100 gm	31 gm
Millet	1 cup	8.5 gm

APPENDIX V

CHARTS

BODY STATISTICS CHART
(Measure in cm for women)

Date ⇒ Body Part ⇓	15/07/13	15/08/13	15/9/13
Calf			
Lower Thigh			
Upper Thigh			
Hip			
Below Navel			
Navel			
Narrowest Circumference of Waist			
Chest			

Date ⇒ Body Part ⇓	15/07/13	15/08/13	15/9/13
Upper Arm			
Lower Arm			
Forearm			
Wrist			
Fat Percentage			
Weight			

GOAL SETTING

Category	Goal	Time Frame	Achievement Status
Cardio			
Strength			

Category	Goal	Time Frame	Achievement Status
Flexibility			
Diet			
Others			

APPENDIX VI

NOTES

AEROBIC EXERCISE

The word aerobic means 'with oxygen'; anaerobic is 'without the supply of oxygen'. Moderate intensity exercise, which utilizes oxygen, is traditionally used to maintain stamina or cardiovascular fitness. Aerobic exercise is the mainstay of any fitness routine. It improves the condition of your heart and lungs (your cardiorespiratory system). Cardiorespiratory endurance is the ability of the body's circulatory and respiratory systems to supply fuel during sustained physical activity (USDHHS, 1996, as adapted from Corbin & Lindsey, 1994).

There are three main processes by which energy is derived for the working of the muscles. ATP or adenosine triphosphate is the main source of energy.

- **Aerobic Metabolism:** When one participates in low to moderate intensity physical exercise, a continuous supply of oxygen helps in the conversion of nutrients like carbohydrates and fats to ATP through what is called the Krebs cycle. This kind of exercise can be continued for prolonged periods of time (2-3 hours), and is primarily sustained by **slow twitch muscle fibres**. Mainly carbohydrates provide for the ATP at this level of exercise. Once the store of carbohydrate is depleted, and if not replenished with a sports drink or any other source, the individual is unable to continue with the exercise due to what appears to be intense fatigue. This is called **hitting the wall**. This is one of the reasons one has to be adequately nourished with easily digestible carbohydrates before a long-duration exercise. Often called **carb loading**, it is practised before marathons and triathlons.

- **Anaerobic Metabolism** provides energy for short-duration intense exercises like sprinting or lifting very heavy weight. There are two systems at work:

  1. The **ATP-CP system**: There are small stores of ready ATP in the muscle cells themselves. The first few seconds of intense exercise will utilize this already available ATP. This store is depleted in about 10 seconds, however, like in the first 10 seconds of a 100-metre sprint.

  2. The **anaerobic glycolysis** then kicks in, creating ATP from glycogen in the absence of oxygen, with lactic acid being the by-product. This metabolic pathway can provide energy through the partial breakdown of glycogen in the muscle for short, intense exercise for approximately 3 minutes before the accumulation of lactic acid occurs within the muscles. At this point, the muscles are said to reach their **lactate threshold**. The pain and intense burning sensation in the muscles make it difficult to continue with the exercise. High Intensity Interval Training or HIIT has been known to improve the body's capacity to facilitate anaerobic glycolysis and increase the lactate threshold. The **fast twitch muscle fibres** seem to be more adept at anaerobic glycolysis. Training at a high intensity at frequent intervals has

been found to increase the number of fast twitch fibres.
(*See chapter 5*)

CRITICISM OF THE SURGEON GENERAL'S STATEMENT

There is some criticism on the surgeon general's statement.
The STRRIDE study (Studies of Targeted Risk Reduction
Intervention through Defined Exercise) was designed to
investigate the effects of different quantities and intensities of
exercise on metabolic risk factors for cardiovascular disease,
diabetes, weight loss, amount of abdominal fat, and so on. An
analysis of some of the results of the study showed that the
recommended 'mandatory minimum requirement', as stated by
the surgeon general, may not be sufficient for people of different
body weights. A woman weighing 150 kg, for instance, may be
able to burn those 150 calories in 15 minutes by the pure merit
of her weight (calorie burn is calculated using the body weight,
time and kind of activity). Does this mean she stops with 15
minutes of exercise? On the other hand, a much fitter woman
weighing only 50 kg may take 30 minutes to burn 150 calories.
So, by definition, the obese woman needs to exercise for 15
minutes while the fitter, leaner woman is required to exercise
for 30 minutes.

One prudent approach would be to recommend that all
adults aim for 30 minutes of moderate intensity activity each
day and then let body weight changes be the broad measure
for determining if this amount of activity is adequate. For
individuals who still gain weight at this activity level without
significant dietary changes, increasing daily activity to 40–45
minutes would be the next step. I argue that this individualized
approach might be an important component of national activity
recommendations that would greatly minimize the confusion
surrounding the surgeon general's normative recommendations

for physical activity levels required to maintain health and wellness. (*See chapter 5*)

TALK TEST

This test has been found to correlate very well with the more complicated evaluation of VO2 Max (maximum oxygen uptake) and target heart rate. (*See chapter 5*)

BIBLIOGRAPHY

American Council on Exercise, *ACE Personal Trainer Manual: The Ultimate Resource for Fitness Professionals* (2010).

American Heart Association, 'Statement on Exercise: Benefits and Recommendations for Physical Activity Programs for all Americans: A Statement for Health Professionals by the Committee on Exercise and Cardiac Rehabilitation of the Council on Clinical Cardiology, American Heart Association', *Circulation*, 86 (1992).

Amen, Daniel G., *The Amen Solution: The Brain Healthy Way to Lose Weight and Keep It Off* (New York, 2011).

Amorim Adegboye, A. R. et al., 'Diet or Exercise, or Both, for Weight Reduction in Women after Childbirth', *Cochrane Database of Systematic Reviews*, 3 (2007).

Andersen, J. L. et al., 'Muscle, Genes and Athletic Performance', *Scientific American Magazine*, (September 2000).

Ayas, Najib T. et al., 'A Prospective Study of Self-Reported Sleep Duration and Incident Diabetes in Women', *Diabetes Care*, 26/2 (2003).

Berek, Jonathan S., *Novac's Gynecology* (New York, 2002).

Bickel, C. S. et al., 'Exercise Dosing to Retain Resistance Training Adaptations in Young and Older Adults', *Medicine and Science in Sports and Exercise*, 43/7 (2011).

Boone, Lena, 'Is Your Workout Making You Sick? A New Level of Overtraining', *Bodybuilding.com*, 2 April 2009.

Bray, G. A., '*Good Calories, Bad Calories* by Gary Taubes; New York: AA Knopf', *Obesity Reviews*, 9 (2008).

Bryant, Cedric X. and Daniel J. Green, eds, *ACE Personal Trainer Manual: The Ultimate Resource for Fitness Professionals* (2003).

Busch, A. J. et al., 'Exercise for Treating Fibromyalgia Syndrome', *Cochrane Database of Systematic Reviews*, 4 (2007).

Carey, V. J. et al., 'Body Fat Distribution and Risk of Non-Insulin-Dependent Diabetes Mellitus in Women. The Nurses' Health Study', *American Journal of Epidemiology*, 145/7 (1997).

Colditz, G. A. and S. E. Hankinson, 'The Nurses' Health Study: Lifestyle and Health among Women', *Nature Reviews Cancer*, 5/5 (2005).

—— —— and J. E. Manson, 'The Nurses' Health Study: 20-Year Contribution to the Understanding of Health among Women', *Journal of Women's Health*, 6/1 (1997).

Cotton, Richard T. and Ross E. Anderson, *Clinical Exercise Specialist Manual: ACE's Source for Training Special Populations* (San Diego, 1999).

Delavier, Frédéric, *Strength Training Anatomy* (France, 2001).

Derenne, Jennifer L. et al., 'Body Image, Media and Eating Disorders', *Academic Psychiatry*, 30 (2006).

Dokken, Betsy B. and Tsu-Shuen Tsao, 'The Physiology of Body Weight Regulation: Are We Too Efficient for Our Own Good?', *Diabetes Spectrum*, 20/3 (2007).

'Effects of Obesity and Exercise: Is Obesity a Mental Health Issue? The Harvard Mental Health Letter Investigates', *Harvard Health Publications* (2004).

Ellis, Albert, *Overcoming Destructive Beliefs, Feelings, and Behaviors* (Amherst, 2001).

Fjeldstad, Cecilie et al., 'Influence of Obesity on Falls and Quality of Life', *Dynamic Medicine*, 7/4 (2008).

Foster, C., 'Monitoring Training in Athletes with Reference to Overtraining Syndrome', *Medicine and Science in Sports and Exercise*, 30/7 (1998).

Fransen, M. et al., 'Exercise for Osteoarthritis of the Knee', *Cochrane Database of Systematic Reviews*, 4 (2008).

Groves, Barry, 'William Banting: The Father of the Low Carbohydrate Diet' (2002).

Grundy, Scott M. et al., 'Diagnosis and Management of the Metabolic Syndrome: An American Heart Association/National Heart, Lung, and Blood Institute Scientific Statement', *Circulation*, 112 (2005).

Gulati, Martha et al., 'The Prognostic Value of a Nomogram for Exercise Capacity in Women', *The New England Journal of Medicine*, 353 (2005).

Hainer, Vojtech et al., 'Fat or Fit: What Is More Important?', *Diabetes Care*, 32 (2009).

Hall, John E. and Arthur C. Guyton, *Guyton and Hall Textbook of Medical Physiology* (Philadelphia, 2011).

Han, A. et al., 'Tai Chi for Treating Rheumatoid Arthritis', *Cochrane Database of Systematic Reviews*, 3 (2004).

Harms, Craig A. et al., 'Sex Differences in Pulmonary Function during Exercise', *Medicine & Science in Sports & Exercise*, 40/4 (2008).

Herbert, R. D. et al., 'Stretching to Prevent or Reduce Muscle Soreness after Exercise', *Cochrane Database of Systematic Reviews*, 7 (2011).

Hodgdon, J. A. and M. B. Beckett, 'Prediction of Percent Body Fat for US Navy Women from Body Circumference and Height' (Naval Health Research Center San Diego, 1984).

Howe, T. E. et al., 'Exercise for Preventing and Treating Osteoporosis in Postmenopausal Women', *Cochrane Database of Systematic Reviews*, 7 (2011).

Howe, T. E. et al., 'Exercise for Improving Balance in Older People', *Cochrane Database of Systematic Reviews*, 11 (2011).

Innes, Kim E. et al., 'Risk Indices Associated with the Insulin Resistance Syndrome, Cardiovascular Disease, and Possible Protection with Yoga: A Systematic Review', *Journal of the American Board of Family Medicine*, 18/6 (2005).

Kolotkin, R. L. et al., 'Quality of Life and Obesity', *Obesity Reviews*, 2/4 (2008).

Landers, Daniel M., 'The Influence of Exercise on Mental Health', *PCPFS Research Digest*, 2/12.

List, E. O. et al., 'Yoyo Dieting *vs.* Obesity: A Longitudinal Analysis of Body Composition, Glucose Metabolism and Lifespan in

Mice Susceptible to Diet-Induced Obesity', *Endocrine Review*, 32 (2011).

Liu, Simin et al., 'Whole-Grain Consumption and Risk of Coronary Heart Disease: Results from Nurses' Health Study', *The American Journal of Clinical Nutrition*, 70/3 (1999).

Luppino, Floriana S. et al., 'Overweight, Obesity and Depression: A Systematic Review and Meta-Analysis of Longitudinal Studies', *Archives of General Psychiatry*, 67/3 (2010).

MacLean, Paul S. et al., 'Regular Exercise Attenuates the Metabolic Drive to Regain Weight after Long-Term Weight Loss', *American Journal of Physiology Regulatory, Integrative and Comparative Physiology*, 297/3 (2009).

MacLean, Paul S. et al., 'Biology's Response to Dieting: the Impetus for Weight Regain', *American Journal of Physiology Regulatory, Integrative and Comparative Physiology*, 301/3 (2011).

Mayhew, J. L. and P. M. Gross, 'Body Composition Changes in Young Women with High Resistance Weight Training', *Research Quarterly*, 45/4 (1974).

McElroy, Susan L. et al., 'Are Mood Disorders and Obesity Related?', *Journal of Clinical Psychiatry*, 65/5 (2004).

Meckling, Kelly A. and Rachel Sherfrey, 'A Randomized Trial of a Hypocaloric High-Protein Diet, with and without Exercise on Weight Loss, Fitness, and Markers of Metabolic Syndrome in Overweight and Obese Women', *Applied Physiology, Nutrition and Metabolism*, 32/4 (2007).

Miller, W. C. et al., 'A Meta-Analysis of the Past 25 Years of Weight Loss Research Using Diet, Exercise or Diet plus Exercise Intervention', *International Journal of Obesity*, 21/10 (1997).

Misra, A. et al., 'Waist Circumference Cutoff Points and Action Levels for Asian Indians for Identification of Abdominal Obesity', *International Journal of Obesity*, 30/1 (2005).

Misra, A. et al., 'Consensus Statement for Diagnosis of Obesity, Abdominal Obesity and the Metabolic Syndrome for Asian Indians and Recommendations for Physical Activity, Medical and Surgical Management', *Journal of the Association of Physicians in India*, 57 (February 2009).

Moran, Lisa J. et al., 'Lifestyle Changes in Women with Polycystic Ovary Syndrome', *Cochrane Database of Systematic Reviews*, 7 (2011).

Oh, Kyungwon et al., 'Dietary Fat Intake and Risk of Coronary Heart Disease in Women: 20 Years of Follow-up of Nurses' Health Study', *American Journal of Epidemiology*, 161/7 (2005).

Orozco, L. J. et al., 'Exercise or Exercise and Diet for Preventing Type 2 Diabetes Mellitus', *Cochrane Database of Systematic Reviews*, 3 (2008).

Oswald, Dr Christopher and Dr Stanley N. Bacso, *Stretching for Fitness, Health & Performance: The Complete Handbook for All Ages and Fitness Levels* (2003).

Penedo, Frank J. and Jason R. Dahn, 'Exercise and Well-Being: A Review of Mental and Physical Health Benefits Associated with Physical Activity', *Current Opinion in Psychiatry*, 18/2 (2005).

Phillips, K. A., 'Body Dysmorphic Disorder: The Distress of Imagined Ugliness', *The American Journal of Psychiatry*, 148/9 (1991).

—— —— and Rocco D. Crino, 'Body Dysmorphic Disorder', *Current Opinion in Psychiatry*, 14/2 (2001).

Ploutz-Snyder, Lori L. and E. L. Gamis, 'Orientation and Familiarization to 1RM Strength Testing in Old and Young Women', *Journal of Strength and Conditioning Research*, 15/4 (2001).

Raman, Dr Krishna, *Yoga & Medical Science: FAQ* (2003).

Rimer, J. et al., 'Exercise for Depression', *Cochrane Database of Systematic Reviews*, 7 (2012).

Ross, Alyson and Sue Thomas, 'The Health Benefits of Yoga and Exercise: A Review of Comparison Studies', *The Journal of Alternative and Complementary Medicine*, 16/1 (2010).

Scheinfeld, N. S. et al., 'A Primer of Skin Diseases Associated with Obesity', *Expert Review of Dermatology*, 2/4 (2007).

Shaw, K. A. et al., 'Psychological Interventions for Overweight or Obesity', *Cochrane Database of Systematic Reviews*, 2 (2005).

Shaw, K. A. et al., 'Exercise for Overweight or Obesity', *Cochrane Database of Systematic Reviews*, 4 (2006).

Shekar, M. A. et al., 'Study of Incidence of Obesity in Newly Diagnosed Type 2 Diabetics Using Anthropometric Measurements', *International Journal of Diabetes in Developing Countries*, 25 (2005).

Singh, Devendra and Robert K. Young, 'Body Weight, Waist-to-Hip Ratio, Breasts, and Hips: Role in Judgments of Female Attractiveness and Desirability for Relationships', *Ethology and Sociobiology*, 16 (1995).

Snehalatha, Chamukuttan et al., 'Cutoff Values for Normal Anthropometric Variables in Asian Indian Adults', *Diabetes Care*, 26/5 (2003).

Stiles, Mukunda, *Structural Yoga Therapy: Adapting to the Individual* (Boston, 2000).

US Department of Health and Human Services, *Physical Activity and Health: A Report of the Surgeon General* (Atlanta, 1996).

Weinsier, Roland L. et al., 'Do Adaptive Changes in Metabolic Rate Favor Weight Regain in Weight-Reduced Individuals? An Examination of the Set-Point Theory', *The American Journal of Clinical Nutrition*, 72/5 (2000).

Wener, W. K. H. and Sharon A. Hoeger, *Principles and Labs for Fitness & Wellness* (Belmont, 2008).

WHO Expert Consultation, 'Appropriate Body-Mass Index for Asian Populations and Its Implications for Policy and Intervention Strategies', *The Lancet*, 363/9403 (2004).

Yagnik, C. S., 'Obesity Epidemic in India: Intrauterine Origins?', *Proceedings of the Nutrition Society*, 63/3 (2004).

—— —— 'Fetal Programming of Diabetes, Still So Much to Learn', *Diabetes Care*, 33/5 (2010).

Zagaria, M.A., 'Sarcopenia: Loss of Muscle Mass in Older Adults', *US Pharmacist*, 35/9 (2010).